MCQs
for Dentistry

Wu 18 JON £17.99

MCQs
for Dentistry

Judith Jones
and
Kathy Fan

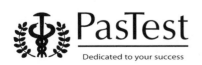

PasTest
Dedicated to your success

© 2006 PASTEST LTD
Egerton Court
Parkgate Estate
Knutsford
Cheshire
WA16 8DX

Telephone: 01565 752000

First Published 2006
ISBN: 1 904627528

A catalogue record for this book is available from the British Library.

The information contained within this book was obtained by the author from reliable sources. However, while every effort has been made to ensure its accuracy, no responsibility for loss, damage or injury occasioned to any person acting or refraining from action as a result of information contained herein can be accepted by the publishers or author.

PasTest Revision Books and Intensive Courses
PasTest has been established in the field of postgraduate medical education since 1972, providing revision books and intensive study courses for doctors preparing for their professional examinations.

Books and courses are available for the following specialties:
MRCGP, MRCP Parts 1 and 2, MRCPCH Parts 1 and 2, MRCPsych, MRCS, MRCOG Parts 1 and 2, DRCOG, DCH, FRCA, PLAB Parts 1 and 2.

For further details contact:
PasTest, Freepost, Knutsford, Cheshire WA16 7BR
Tel: 01565 752000 Fax: 01565 650264
www.pastest.co.uk enquiries@pastest.co.uk

Text prepared by Carnegie Book Production, Lancaster
Printed and bound in the UK by Page Bros Ltd, Norwich

Contents

List of Contributors

Julia Costello BDS MSc
Clinical Demonstrator, Department of Periodontology
Guy's Hospital, Kings College London

Mandeep Ghuman BDS BSc(Hons) MFDS RCS (Eng)
Senior House Officer
Kent & Canterbury Hospital
Canterbury, Kent

Introduction

Multiple choice questions have been used for many years as a way of testing a candidate's knowledge and recall of information. Over the years, they have been in and out of vogue but a lot of courses have seen a resurgence in their usage recently. The cynics amongst you may think that MCQs are popular because they are easy to mark. Whatever the reason, they are an accepted and frequently used method of testing knowledge.

The MCQs in this book are of the "true/false" variety. The questions will start with a statement or stem followed by a group of phrases. You need to mark each statement as to whether you think it is true or false. Each phrase is independent of the others in the group and there can be any combination of true and false phrases in a question.

The aim is to get as many marks as possible so it is necessary to know how the questions are going to be marked. For example, if negative marking is used then you receive a mark for each correct answer and have a mark deducted for each wrong answer. This is important to know as guessing in this type of test will cause you to lose marks. However, if there is no negative marking it is possible to guess answers without losing marks.

When doing MCQs, it is important to read the questions carefully and read what is written and not what you expect to read. For example, there are often little things in them to trip you up like double negatives. Rest assured, we have tried not to incorporate them in the questions in this book. Another tip is to look for questions that include words like "always" and "never" as these are often false. Each question usually has the same amount of marks so it is important to do the whole paper.

As with most things, the only way to get good at MCQs is to practise them and this book will provide you with an opportunity to do that. Each question has the true answers listed on the following page and a short explanation about the questions to help your revision.

This book is intended to help you practise MCQs to prepare for examinations in dentistry and is suitable for both undergraduates and postgraduates students. We hope you find it useful and wish you every success in your forthcoming examinations.

Judith Jones & Kathy Fan

1

General
Dentistry

1.1 **At which of the following autoclave conditions would sterilisation be achieved?**

A   121 °C for 15 minutes

B   121 °C for 5 minutes

C   121 °C for 3 minutes

D   134 °C for 3 minutes

E   134 °C for 5 minutes

1.2 **Which of the following requirements must be satisfied when gaining informed consent from a patient?**

A   The patient has a chaperone

B   The consent is voluntary

C   A written list of warnings must be given to the patient

D   The patient understands the treatment plan

E   The patient is over 18 years of age

1.3 **Which of the following are responsibilities of the General Dental Council?**

A   Registration of dentists

B   Registration of dental practices

C   Protection of the public

D   Professional indemnity

E   Ensuring continuing professional development

1.1 ADE

Recommended autoclave cycles are usually 121 °C for 15 minutes or 134 °C for 3 minutes. Sterilisation will also be achieved at 134 °C for 5 minutes but is not necessary as it is already achieved at 3 minutes at this temperature.

1.2 BD

Consent can only be gained when the procedure, the consequences of not carrying out the procedure and alternative treatments have been explained to the patient. All the risks, complications and benefits of the procedure must be explained, and the patient should understand the information given. Consent must be voluntary. Patients under 16 years of age may give consent for treatment provided they understand the above conditions (Gillick competence).

1.3 ACE

The General Dental Council is the regulatory body of the dental profession. It protects the public by means of its statutory responsibility for registration, dental education and professional conduct and health. It also supports dentists in the practice of dentistry and encourages their continuing professional development.

1.4 **Which of the following protocols must be included in the 'written practice protocols'?**

A Disposal of hazardous waste

B Disposal of sharps

C Annual leave entitlements

D Radiation protection

E Autoclaving

1.5 **Who may be given access to a patient's dental records without their permission?**

A The patient's spouse/partner

B The patient's employer

C An insurance/defence organisation if it is investigating an allegation of negligence

D A court of law

E The patient's parents

1.6 **Which of the following conditions must be met in order to prove dental negligence?**

A The patient was not happy with the treatment as it was of a poor standard

B The dentist had a duty of care to the patient

C The patient was overcharged for the treatment

D Duty of care was breached

E Breach of care resulted in damage

1.4   ABDE

Written practice protocols should include information on radiation protection, cleaning and sterilization of instruments and impressions, disposal of sharps and hazardous waste, protective clothing and medical history forms.

1.5   CD

Confidentiality is almost always absolute. However, there are a few circumstances when patient information may be passed on. For example, records may be passed to other healthcare professionals treating the patient or to an insurance company/defence organisation in relation to a claim. Occasionally there may be a legal requirement, for example to disclose information to a court of law or if there is a notifiable infectious disease. In addition, dental records may have to be released for the purpose of identifying missing persons.

1.6   BDE

In order for a claimant (or patient) to prove that a dentist was negligent they must prove that the dentist had a duty of care which was breached and that this resulted in harm or injury.

1.7 **Which of the following statements about fluoride are true?**

A   Fluoride has an effect on enamel only if it is given while the tooth is forming

B   Fluoride is absorbed mainly from the duodenum and is excreted by the kidneys

C   Fluoride is absorbed mainly from the stomach and is excreted by the kidneys

D   Fluoride is more effective at decreasing pit and fissure caries than smooth surface caries

E   Fluoride is more effective at decreasing smooth surface caries than pit and fissure caries

1.8 **Which of the following cross-infection control measures should be adopted by all dental personnel?**

A   Immunisation against hepatitis B

B   Immunisation against hepatitis C

C   Immunisation against hepatitis A

D   Wearing of gloves when treating patients

E   Wearing of eye protection

1.9 **Which of the following are known to be risk factors for oral cancer?**

A   Tobacco consumption

B   Social deprivation

C   Alcohol consumption

D   High levels of stress

E   Previous trauma to the site

1.7   CE

Fluoride has an effect on enamel both while the tooth is forming and after eruption. It is absorbed from the stomach and excreted via the kidneys.

1.8   ADE

Universal cross-infection control measures should be taken when treating all patients. These include immunisation against hepatitis B and wearing gloves, masks and eye protection as well as protective clothing. At present there is no vaccination available against hepatitis C. Hepatitis A is a viral infection that is spread via the oro-faecal route, and is unlikely to be transmitted by dental treatment, especially where universal precautions are employed.

1.9   ABC

Risk factors for oral cancer include tobacco smoking, tobacco chewing, snuff usage, betel nut chewing, alcohol consumption and social deprivation. Previous trauma and stress are not thought to have an effect.

1.10 **Which of the following foodstuffs/drinks contain fluoride not added by the manufacturer/supplier?**

A Coffee

B Tea

C Salt

D Bony fish

E Wine

1.11 **Deposition of local anaesthetic solution close to the left lingula of the mandible is likely to anaesthetise the:**

A Left side of the anterior aspect of the tongue

B Labial gingivae on the left

C Buccal gingivae of the left lower molars

D Left side of the posterior third of the tongue

E Pulp of the lower molars on the left

1.12 **Clinical records for adults should be kept for:**

A 3 years

B 5 years

C 7 years

D 11 years

E 15 years

1.10 BD

Bony fish, tea and beer contain naturally occurring fluoride.

1.11 ABE

Depositing local anaesthetic in the region of the left lingula will anaesthetise the left inferior dental nerve, and hence the pulps of the lower teeth and the labial gingivae on the left will go numb. As the lingual nerve lies close to the lingula it is also possible to anaethetise it, so the left side of the anterior aspect of the tongue will go numb. The posterior aspect of the tongue is supplied by the glossopharyngeal and vagus nerves. The long buccal nerve supplies the buccal gingivae of the lower molars.

1.12 D

All clinical records should be kept for 11 years for adults. For children, clinical records should be kept until the individual is 25 years old or for 11 years, whichever is longer.

1.13 If a person has undergone a course of vaccination against the hepatitis B virus, which of the following antibody levels would imply that they have responded to the vaccination and are protected against catching the infection?

A   HbsAb > 1 mIU/ml

B   HbsAb > 10 mIU/ml

C   HbsAb > 100 mIU/ml

D   HbsAg > 1000 mIU/ml

E   None of the above

1.14 Which of the following are essential features of cariogenic bacteria:

A   Ability to attach to the smooth surface of a tooth

B   Ability to produce acid with an appropriate pH (pH > 6) to decalcify tooth substance

C   Ability to survive in stagnant areas

D   Ability to form insoluble glucans

E   Ability to metabolise sugar alcohols (polyols)

1.15 Dental hygienists are allowed to:

A   Record periodontal probing depths

B   Record mobility of teeth

C   Give oral hygiene instruction

D   Give inferior dental nerve blocks under supervision

E   Take dental impressions

1.13   CD

Protection against hepatitis B usually occurs with HbsAg antibody levels greater than 100 mIU/ml.

1.14   AD

The bacteria need to be able to produce enough acid so that the pH drops to < 5. The cariogenicity of *Streptococcus mutans* stems from its ability to produce large amounts of insoluble glucans (to enable adhesion) and acid. Sugar alcohols are non-cariogenic, eg sorbitol.

1.15   ABC

Hygienists may only work under the supervision of a registered dentist and the treatment plan must be written down and less than a year old. They are allowed to record probing depths and tooth mobility, and give oral hygiene instruction. They should not take impressions or give inferior dental nerve blocks, even under supervision.

1.16 **With respect to continuing professional development (CPD), a dentist must carry out:**

A   75 hours of CPD of which 25 must be certifiable over a year

B   150 hours of CPD of which 50 must be certifiable over a year

C   200 hours of CPD of which 75 must be certifiable over a 5-year period

D   250 hours of CPD of which 75 must be certifiable over a 5-year period

E   CPD is left up to the individual dentist's needs

1.17 **With regard to dental nomenclature systems:**

A   An upper right first permanent molar may be written as 26 using the World Dental Federation (FDI) system

B   An upper right first permanent molar may be written as 16 using the FDI system

C   A lower left deciduous canine may be written as 33 using the FDI system

D   A lower left deciduous canine may be written as 43 using the FDI system

E   A lower left deciduous canine may be written as 3C using the FDI system

1.18 **When disposing of waste from a dental practice, it is important to separate waste into the appropriate category for disposal (clinical, non-clinical and special waste). Which of the following are examples of special waste?**

A   Blood-stained gauze

B   Radiography fixer solution

C   Alginate impression

D   Half a cartridge of 2% lidocaine and 1:80 000 adrenaline

E   Mercury

1.16   D

'CPD' means studying, training, attending courses and seminars, reading and other activities undertaken by a dentist, which could reasonably be expected to advance their professional development as a dentist. CPD is mandatory for all registered dentists. A 'CPD cycle' is a 5-year period and dentists must complete 250 hours of CPD of which 75 hours are verifiable. Dentists should keep up-to-date records of the CPD that they undertake and submit these to the General Dental Council on demand.

1.17   B

The quadrants are numbered as follows:

- Upper right permanent – 1
- Upper left permanent – 2
- Lower left permanent – 3
- Lower right permanent – 4
- Upper right deciduous – 5
- Upper left deciduous – 6
- Lower left deciduous – 7
- Lower right deciduous – 8

Permanent and deciduous teeth are numbered 1–8 and 1–5, respectively, in each quadrant starting from the midline. Hence the upper right first permanent molar would be written as 16 and the lower left deciduous canine would be written as 73.

1.18 BDE

All mercury waste and radiography developer and fixative solutions must be disposed of as special waste, as must all prescribed medicines. As local anaesthetic is in effect a prescribed medicine it is treated as special waste. Anything contaminated with body fluids should be disposed off in the clinical waste, eg impressions and blood-stained gauze.

2

Human
Disease

2.1   **Which of the following conditions might make a patient susceptible to infective endocarditis following dental treatment?**

    A   Previous history of rheumatic fever

    B   Presence of a cardiac pacemaker

    C   Congenital cardiac lesion

    D   Diagnosis of atrial fibrillation

    E   Heart murmur

2.2   **A patient tells you that they have had hepatitis. Which of the following may be of concern when providing dental treatment for them?**

    A   The patient will need antibiotic cover for invasive procedures

    B   Increased bleeding following invasive procedures due to impaired synthesis of clotting factors

    C   High risk of infective endocarditis after extractions

    D   Possible cross-infection risk

    E   Impaired drug metabolism

2.3   **A patient gives a history of rheumatic fever. Which of the following procedures require prophylactic antibiotic cover?**

    A   Scale and polish

    B   Extraction of a tooth

    C   Inferior dental nerve block

    D   Impression for a new lower complete denture

    E   Placing a class I amalgam restoration

2.1 ACE

Patients who have valvular defects that are either congenital in origin or due to rheumatic fever, patients with congenital cardiac defects, eg ventricular septal defects, and patients with aortic regurgitation, mitral regurgitation or aortic stenosis are at risk of infective endocarditis following a bacteraemia. Hence, they require prophylactic antibiotic cover. Patients with cardiac pacemakers or atrial fibrillation do not require prophylactic antibiotic cover.

Note: The complete list of the types of cardiac lesion requiring antibiotic cover is freely available from the British Cardiac Society website (www.bcs.com).

2.2 BDE

Patients with liver disease are likely to have disordered clotting and abnormal drug metabolism. If their disease is due to infective hepatitis there may be a risk of cross-infection. Prophylactic antibiotic cover is not required for patients with liver disease, nor are they susceptible to infective endocarditis following extractions.

2.3 AB

Antibiotic cover is required for all procedures likely to cause bacteraemia. These include scaling, polishing and extractions.

2.4 **Which of the following statements about Down's syndrome are true?**

A It is caused by trisomy 20

B It is caused by trisomy 21

C The incidence increases with increasing age of the mother

D Patients with Down's syndrome often have delayed eruption of teeth

E Patients with Down's syndrome often have microglossia

F Patients with Down's syndrome often have congenital cardiac defects

2.5 **Which of the following statements regarding the Resuscitation Council's (UK) recommendations of the ratio of compressions to breaths per minute are/is correct?**

A Depends on the number of rescuers

B Use a ratio of 30 compressions to 2 rescue breaths if there are two rescuers

C Use a ratio of 15 compressions to 2 rescue breaths if there is one rescuer

D Use a ratio of 5 compressions to 1 rescue breath if there are two rescuers

E Use a ratio of 5 compressions to 1 rescue breath if there is one rescuer

2.6 **Which of the following are recommended by the Resuscitation Council (UK) when performing basic life support on an adult?**

A Ensure safety of rescuer and victim

B If victim is not breathing, give two slow, effective rescue breaths and then go for help if you are alone

C Look, listen and feel for 20 seconds to determine if the victim is breathing normally

D Assess the victim for signs of circulation by checking the radial pulse

E If there are no signs of circulation, start external cardiac compression by applying pressure over the left side of the chest

2.4   BCDF

Down's syndrome is a condition caused by trisomy 21. Its incidence increases with increasing age of the mother. Patients often have delayed eruption of teeth, macroglossia and congenital cardiac lesions, which require prophylactic antibiotic cover for invasive dental procedures.

2.5   B

Current Resuscitation Council (UK) guidelines advise using the same ratio for both one and two rescuers. The aim is 100 compressions per minute, and 30 compressions to 2 rescue breaths. New guidelines were published at the end of 2005, with changed compression : breath ratio (see www.resus.org.uk).

2.6   A

The first priority is safety and so the rescuer should be aware of any potential risks associated with attempting to resuscitate a victim and these risks should be eliminated or minimised prior to attempting resuscitation. If the victim is not breathing or is only making occasional gasps or weak attempts at breathing, send someone for help. If you are on your own, leave the victim and go for assistance.

Assess the circulation by looking, listening and feeling for normal breathing, coughing or movement by the victim, and check the carotid pulse within 10 seconds if trained to do so. The radial pulse is not used to assess the circulation in this situation. External cardiac compression is performed by pressing over the middle of victim's chest and not on the left side.

2.7 **A patient complains of severe chest pain while in your dental chair. Appropriate management includes:**

A Lie the patient flat

B Lie the patient in the recovery position

C Administer sublingual glyceryl trinitrate (GTN)

D Give the patient oxygen

E Administer Hypostop® gel buccally

2.8 **You have a patient with known diabetes who becomes sweaty in the dental chair. How would you manage this situation?**

A Continue with what you are doing and aim to finish quickly

B Check if the patient had eaten and give them some glucose

C Check if the patient had eaten and give them some insulin

D Check their blood glucose (BM)

E Try to calm the patient as they are probably anxious

2.9 **Anaphylaxis:**

A Is caused by an acute-type intravenous allergic response

B Results in acute hypertension, bronchospasm and urticaria

C Is managed by laying the patient flat and maintaining the airway

D Is managed by giving 0.5 ml of 1:1000 adrenaline (epinephrine) intravenously

E Is managed by giving oxygen

2.7 CD

Lying the patient flat may make their breathing more difficult, so this is not advised. Sublingual GTN can be given as the pain may be due to angina. Hypostop® gel is a glucose-containing gel that is used in hypoglycaemic events.

2.8 BD

Diabetic patients could forget to eat prior to their appointment and may be hypoglycaemic. If there is doubt whether the patient has hypo/hyperglycaemia it is safer to give the patient glucose as it will do no immediate harm to the hyperglycaemic patient but may save the hypoglycaemic patient.

If there are signs that the patient is not well, it is always best to abort the procedure and deal with the medical issues.

2.9 CE

Anaphylaxis is caused by a type I hypersensitivity reaction during which histamine is released from mast cells. This causes acute hypotension, bronchospasm and urticaria. Management involves laying the patient flat, maintaining the airway and giving drugs including 0.5 ml of 1:1000 adrenaline (epinephrine) intramuscularly and oxygen.

2.10 Which of the following is recommended by the Resuscitation Council (UK)?

A A ratio of 5 breaths to 1 compression when a single person is carrying out basic life support (BLS)

B A ratio of 5 breaths to 1 compression when two people are carrying out BLS

C A ratio of 15 breaths to 2 compressions when a single person is carrying out BLS

D A ratio of 15 breaths to 2 compressions when two people are carrying out BLS

E A ratio of 30 breaths to 1 compression at all times

2.11 With regard to the following emergencies, which commonly used drugs and doses are correct?

A Anaphylaxis – 0.5 ml of 1:100 adrenaline (epinephrine) solution intramuscularly

B Anaphylaxis – 10–20 mg chlorphenamine intravenously

C Diabetic collapse – 20 units of insulin subcutaneously

D Steroid collapse – 100–200 mg hydrocortisone sodium succinate intravenously

E Diabetic collapse – 10 mg glucagon intramuscularly

2.12 The following sites are frequently used for intramuscular injections:

A Vastus lateralis

B Deltoid

C Gluteal muscle

D Antecubital fossa

E Dorsum of the hand

2.10   All statements are false

The Resuscitation Council (UK) recommends 30 compressions to 2 breaths for BLS whether one or two people are carrying it out.

2.11   BD

In anaphylaxis, 0.5 ml of 1:1000 adrenaline (epinephrine) solution is given intramuscularly and 10–20 mg intravenous chlorphenamine is also used. In a diabetic collapse, insulin should never be given in an emergency situation. It is only used when the blood glucose level is known. Glucagon 1 mg intramuscularly can be given.

2.12   ABC

There are eight possible sites where intramuscular injections can be given, four on either side of the body: vastus lateralis muscle (thigh), deltoid muscle (upper arm), and ventrogluteal and dorsal gluteal muscles.

2.13 Pregnant women:

A Can present with an epulis

B Rarely get gingivitis

C May become hypotensive when supine

D Can take aspirin safely

E Must always be given prilocaine (Citanest) and felypressin as a local anaesthetic

2.14 Patients with which of the following conditions/drug treatment regimens may be at risk of an addisonian crisis?

A Addison's disease

B Diabetes insipidus

C Secondary hypoadrenalism

D Long-term steroid therapy

E Cushing's disease

2.15 Diabetic patients:

A Have reduced resistance to dental infection

B Have faster healing following surgery

C May have accelerated periodontal disease

D Are more prone to dental cysts

E Should not be given lidocaine and adrenaline as a local anaesthetic

2.13 AC

In late pregnancy, some patients become hypotensive when supine as the pregnant uterus impedes venous return. Pregnant ladies often get gingivitis. Aspirin is best avoided in pregnancy as it can delay onset and increase duration of labour and increase blood loss, as well as causing premature closure of the fetal ductus arteriosus. Pregnant women can be given lidocaine and adrenaline perfectly safely.

2.14 ACD

Addisonian crisis is likely to present either in patients on long-term steroids or in those with Addison's disease (primary hypoadrenalism) or secondary aldosteronism. The hypothalamic–pituitary–adrenal axis is suppressed or completely atrophies and cannot respond to additional demand. Adrenal insufficiency has an insidious presentation but may present as an emergency (addisonian crisis) with vomiting, abdominal pain, profound weakness and hypovolaemic shock.

Diabetes insipidus occurs due to either impaired vasopressin secretion or resistance to its action. This leads to polyuria, nocturia and polydipsia. Cushing's disease is characterised by excess glucocorticoid secretion resulting from inappropriate adrenocorticotropic hormone (ACTH) secretion from the pituitary.

2.15 AC

Diabetic patients have reduced resistance to infections and hence are more prone to periodontal disease. They have a slower rate of healing. They are not more prone to dental cysts and can be given lidocaine and adrenaline safely.

2.16 **Which of the following measures are appropriate for managing a patient experiencing an addisonian crisis?**

A   Place the patient in a horizontal position

B   Give glucagon

C   Give intravenous hydrocortisone

D   Set up intravenous infusion of fluid

E   Call for medical assistance

2.17 **Hb 9.5 g/dL, WBC 5.3 x 10^9/l, platelets 200 x 10^9/l, RBC 4.7 x 10^9/l, MCV 76 fl, MCH 21.8 pg. This blood film:**

A   Is consistent with anaemia

B   Shows microcytic anaemia

C   Shows macrocytic anaemia

D   Is consistent with iron deficiency anaemia

E   Is consistent with vitamin B_{12} deficiency anaemia

2.18 **Features of Paget's disease include:**

A   Hypercementosis of teeth, which causes difficulties when extractions are needed

B   Alveolar ridges may increase in size, so that new dentures need to be made

C   Radiographs of bone may show radiolucent areas along with sclerotic areas

D   Patients may suffer from symptoms of compression of cranial nerves

E   Development of osteosarcoma is a common consequence of Paget's disease

2.16 ACDE

Glucagon is given to diabetic patients experiencing hypoglycaemia. Placing the patient supine helps management of shock but watch out if the patient is vomiting.

2.17 ABD

Normal range of values

- Haemoglobin: 8.1–11.2 g/dL [mmol/l] (13.5–18.0 g/dL) (male); 7.4–9.9 g/dL [mmol/l] (11.5–16.0 g/dL) (female)
- WBC: $4–11 \times 10^9/l$
- Platelets: $150–400 \times 10^9/l$
- RBC: $3.8–4.8 \times 10^{12}/l$
- MCV: 80–100 fl (femtolitres)
- MCH: 27–32 pg (picograms)

Anaemia is decreased level of haemoglobin (Hb) in the blood. The features of various types of anaemia are shown in the table below.

	Type of anaemia		
	Microcytic, hypochromic	Normocytic/ normochromic	Macrocytic
Blood film findings	Low MCV; low MCH	Normal MCV and MCH	High MCV
Causes	Iron deficiency Thalassaemia Sideroblastic anaemia	Acute blood loss Anaemia of chronic disease	Vitamin B_{12} deficiency Folate deficiency

2.18 ABCD

Paget's disease is characterised by excessive osteoclastic bone resorption followed by disordered osteoblastic activity, leading to abundant new bone formation which is structurally weak and abnormal. Radiographs reveal radiolucencies and sclerotic areas, and there is also hypercementosis. Bone deposition may lead to compression of the cranial nerves as well as changes in the size and shape of the alveolar ridges. Osteogenic sarcoma is a complication, but it is rare.

2.19 Patients with which of the following conditions may be on long-term anticoagulants?

A   Atrial fibrillation

B   Previous deep vein thrombosis

C   Cardiac pacemakers

D   Prosthetic heart valves

E   Ventricular fibrillation

2.20 A patient starts fitting in your dental chair. Appropriate management options include:

A   Call for the emergency services immediately

B   Protect the patient from harm

C   Place a bite prop in the mouth to prevent the patient from biting the tongue

D   Give 0.5 ml of 1:1000 solution of adrenaline (epinephrine) intramuscularly

E   If the fitting does not stop after 5 minutes give 10–20 mg diazepam

2.21 A patient who weighs 60 kg and is 1 m 50 cm in height would have the following body mass index (BMI):

A   20

B   24

C   28

D   32

E   36

2.19 ABD

Patients with atrial fibrillation, prosthetic heart valves and a history of deep vein thrombosis are treated with long-term anticoagulants. Patients with cardiac pacemakers are not given anticoagulants. Ventricular fibrillation is not compatible with life – it is a condition that results in no cardiac output and occurs in a cardiac arrest situation.

2.20 BE

Most fits can be managed in the dental surgery without calling the emergency services. If the fitting does not stop then assistance should be sought, and diazepam, if available, should be given. It is important to prevent the patient from hurting themselves, which would mean moving loose equipment out of the way. Do not try to put anything in the patient's mouth as they may bite you. Adrenaline is not indicated – it is used in anaphylaxis.

2.21 B

BMI is weight (in kg) squared divided by height (in cm). Hence this patient would have a BMI of 24.

2.22 The patient in Q 2.21 would be classified as:

A Underweight

B Normal

C Overweight

D Obese

E Severely obese

2.23 Anaemia:

A Is defined as haemoglobin level below 11.5 g/dl in females and 13.5 g/dl in males

B Due to iron deficiency is usually macrocytic

C Due to folate deficiency is usually microcytic

D Can be easily assessed by looking at a patient's skin colour

E May occur in sickle cell disease

2.24 Which of the following are fat-soluble vitamins?

A Vitamin B_1

B Vitamin A

C Vitamin C

D Vitamin E

E Vitamin D

2.22 B

The different categories of BMI are shown in the table below

BMI	Description
<20	Underweight
20-25	Normal weight
25-30	Overweight
30-40	Obese
>40	Severely obese

Hence the patient in Q 2.21 would be described as having normal weight.

2.23 AE

Macrocytic anaemia is usually due to vitamin B_{12} or folate deficiency. Microcytic anaemia is usually due to iron deficiency. Skin pallor does not give a good indication of whether a person is anaemic or not. Conjunctival or mucosal pallor gives a better idea, although neither is an accurate way of measuring anaemia. Anaemia may occur in sickle cell disease.

2.24 BDE

Vitamins A, D and E are all fat soluble.

2.25 **Regarding vitamin deficiency:**

A   Vitamin A deficiency causes scurvy

B   Vitamin C deficiency causes beri beri

C   Vitamin D deficiency results in skeletal decalcification

D   Vitamin D deficiency in children causes rickets

E   Vitamin D deficiency in children causes delayed tooth eruption

2.26 **Which of the following are causes of finger clubbing?**

A   Bacterial endocarditis

B   Bronchial carcinoma

C   Congenital cyanotic cardiac disease

D   Angina

E   Chronic pulmonary suppuration

2.27 **Features of bacterial endocarditis include:**

A   Boutonniére's deformity

B   Night sweats

C   History of recent dental extractions

D   Splinter haemorrhages

E   Finger clubbing

2.25 CDE

Vitamin C deficiency causes scurvy and vitamin A deficiency results in hyperkeratosis of the skin and visual problems. Beri beri is caused by thiamine (vitamin B_1) deficiency. Vitamin D deficiency causes skeletal problems including decalcification, which in children results in rickets and delayed tooth eruption.

2.26 ABCE

Finger clubbing is the term used to describe fingers where the nail is curved and there is a loss of the angle between the nail and the bed. It occurs in a variety of conditions including: cyanotic cardiac disease; bacterial endocarditis; bronchial carcinoma; liver cirrhosis; ulcerative colitis; conditions with intrathoracic pus, (eg empyema, bronchiectasis); oesophageal ulcers; and Hodgkin's disease. It does not occur in angina.

2.27 BCDE

Infective endocarditis (subacute bacterial endocarditis) is an infection of the endocardium or valvular endothelium of the heart. Clinical features include:

- Infection – fever, night sweats, weight loss and anaemia, splenomegaly, clubbing
- Valve destruction – changing heart murmur leading to heart failure
- Embolic phenomena, eg stroke
- Immune complex deposition – splinter haemorrhages, Roth's spots, Osler's nodes

Boutonniére's deformity of the fingers is seen in rheumatoid arthritis.

2.28 Causes of hypertension include:

A   Conn's syndrome

B   Crohn's disease

C   Phaeochromocytoma

D   Chronic glomerulonephritis

E   Unknown

2.29 Which of the following are concerns in patients who have undergone a transplant?

A   Reduced resistance to infection

B   Xerostomia

C   Caries

D   Susceptibility to osteoradionecrosis following tooth extraction

E   Bleeding tendency

2.30 With respect to bleeding disorders:

A   The prothrombin time is normal in patients with haemophilia

B   The activated partial thromboplastin time is normal in haemophilia A

C   Haemophilia A affects women more frequently than men

D   Haemophilia A is due to factor IX deficiency

E   Bleeding due to von Willebrand's disease may be treated with desmopressin and factor VIII concentrate

2.28 ACDE

In more than 90% of cases of hypertension the cause is unknown. This is referred to as 'essential hypertension'. Secondary hypertension may be due to: renal disease; endocrine disease including Cushing's syndrome, phaeochromocytoma and acromegaly; coarctation of the aorta; pre-eclampsia; and drugs. Conn's syndrome is primary hyperaldosteronism, which causes hypokalaemia and hypernatraemia with hypertension.

2.29 AE

Patients on immunosuppressive drugs are more prone to infections. Bleeding tendencies can occur in renal transplant patients and those with deranged liver function.

2.30 AE

The activated partial thromboplastin time is increased in haemophilia A. Haemophilia A is inherited as an X-linked recessive disease. It affects 1:5000 males and is the result of factor VIII deficiency.

2.31 **Risk factors for ischaemic heart disease that may be modified by the patient include:**

A   Smoking

B   Hypotension

C   Lack of exercise

D   Hypercholesterolaemia

E   Gender

2.32 **Patients with Down's syndrome have:**

A   Macroglossia

B   Periodontal disease

C   Mouth ulcers

D   Delayed tooth eruption

E   Large pulp chambers

2.33 **Which of the following put patients at greater risk of deep vein thrombosis (DVT)?**

A   Being overweight

B   Being on the oral contraceptive pill

C   Early mobilisation following surgery

D   Trauma to a vessel wall

E   Thrombophlebitis

2.31 ACD

Smoking, lack of exercise and hypercholesterolaemia are all risk factors for ischaemic heart disease that a patient could alter. Being male puts a patient at greater risk of ischaemic heart disease, but is not controlled by the patient. Hypertension, not hypotension, is a risk factor.

2.32 ABD

Other features seen in Down's syndrome include: anterior open bite, maxillary hypoplasia, hypodontia, scrotal tongue, and cheilitis. Large pulp chambers are seen in hypophosphataemia.

2.33 ABDE

Risk factors for DVT include being overweight, taking the oral contraceptive pill, thrombophlebitis and trauma to a vessel wall. Early mobilisation after surgery reduces the risk of DVT.

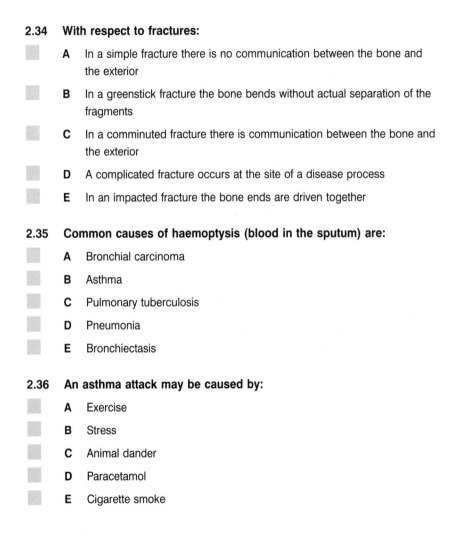

2.34 **With respect to fractures:**

A In a simple fracture there is no communication between the bone and the exterior

B In a greenstick fracture the bone bends without actual separation of the fragments

C In a comminuted fracture there is communication between the bone and the exterior

D A complicated fracture occurs at the site of a disease process

E In an impacted fracture the bone ends are driven together

2.35 **Common causes of haemoptysis (blood in the sputum) are:**

A Bronchial carcinoma

B Asthma

C Pulmonary tuberculosis

D Pneumonia

E Bronchiectasis

2.36 **An asthma attack may be caused by:**

A Exercise

B Stress

C Animal dander

D Paracetamol

E Cigarette smoke

2.34 ABE

A comminuted fracture is one in which there are multiple segments of bone. A complicated fracture is one involving a vital structure, eg a fractured angle of the mandible involving the inferior dental nerve. A pathological fracture occurs at a disease site.

2.35 ACDE

Haemoptysis occurs in pneumonia, tuberculosis, bronchiectasis, bronchial carcinoma and mitral stenosis. It is not a usual feature of asthma.

2.36 ABCE

Common precipitating factors of asthma attacks are exercise, stress, cold weather, fumes, animal dander, cigarette smoke, infections and some drugs, eg propranolol, non-steroidal anti-inflammatory drugs (NSAIDs). Paracetamol does not usually precipitate asthma attacks.

2.37 Regarding the thyroid gland:

A Thyroid hormones increase the metabolism of the body

B In Hashimoto's disease there is autoimmune destruction of the thyroid gland

C Graves' disease is a type of hypothyroidism

D Patients who are hypothyroid often have lethargy, cold intolerance and dry hair

E Patients who are hyperthyroid often have breathlessness, palpitations, increased pulse rate and constipation

2.38 Typical features of an anaphylactic attack include:

A Itching

B Paraesthesia

C Facial flushing

D Bronchodilation

E Hypertension

2.39 Regarding malignant disease:

A Hodgkin's disease is a type of leukaemia

B Acute leukaemia is a common childhood malignancy

C Patients with leukaemia often have intra-oral bleeding

D Patients with multiple myeloma often suffer from bone lesions and pain

E Oral squamous cell carcinomas are usually treated with chemotherapy

2.37 ABD

Graves' disease is a type of hyperthyroidism. Hyperthyroid patients often have breathlessness, palpitations, increased pulse rate and frequent bowel movements.

2.38 ABC

The following signs and symptoms may occur during anaphylactic attacks: facial flushing, itching and paraesthesia, facial oedema, bronchoconstriction, hypotension, pallor, clammy skin, loss of consciousness, rapid pulse and death if adequate treatment is not administered.

2.39 BCD

Hodgkin's disease is a type of lymphoma in which lymphatic tissue is affected, often initially in the neck. Acute leukaemias account for about half of all childhood malignant diseases. Patients with leukaemias often have bleeding tendencies and increased susceptibility to infections; hence they often have bleeding gingivae. Multiple myeloma is a disseminated disease and neoplastic cells are deposited in bone marrow, accounting for the bone pain. Oral squamous cell carcinomas are usually treated with surgery and radiotherapy either independently or in combination. They are usually not treated with chemotherapy alone.

3

Oral
Medicine

3.1   **Which of the following conditions are associated with a known increased risk of malignant change?**

A   Geographic tongue

B   Hairy leukoplakia

C   Sublingual keratosis

D   Denture stomatitis

E   Erosive lichen planus

3.2   **A patient presents with a sore mouth. Which haematological tests would you request?**

A   Full blood count (FBC)

B   Serum ferritin

C   Alkaline phosphatase levels

D   Urea and electrolytes (U&Es)

E   Mean corpuscular volume (MCV)

3.3   **Which of the following are signs of primary herpetic gingivostomatitis?**

A   Dry mouth

B   Intra-oral vesicles

C   Labial vesicles

D   Intra-oral ulcers

E   Low haemoglobin

3.1   CE

Sublingual keratosis has a higher rate of malignant transformation than normal mucosa, as does erosive lichen planus. All the other conditions do not have a higher rate of malignant change.

3.2   ABE

A sore mouth may be due to haematological deficiency and hence blood tests are indicated when a patient complains of a sore mouth. FBC is indicated to determine if the patient is anaemic. The anaemic may be secondary to iron, folate or vitamin B_{12} deficiency. MCV is indicated to determine if the anaemia is microcytic (eg iron deficiency) or macrocytic (B_{12} or folate deficiency).

3.3   BD

Primary herpetic gingivostomatitis is a viral infection caused by the herpes simplex virus. It is usually a subclinical infection. Patients have vesicles that may occur on any part of the oral mucosa, which burst leaving ulcers. Dry mouth and low haemoglobin are not usually seen in this condition. Labial vesicles are seen in recurrent herpes simplex infections.

3.4 **Which of the following are used to treat patients with primary herpetic gingivostomatitis?**

A   A broad-spectrum antibiotic

B   Analgesics

C   An anti-fungal medication

D   Fluids

E   Aciclovir

3.5 **Which of the following are features of secondary Sjögren's syndrome?**

A   Dry mouth (xerostomia)

B   Anosmia (loss of smell)

C   Connective tissue disease

D   Dry eyes (xerophthalmia)

E   Increased incidence of oral squamous cell carcinoma (SCC)

3.6 **Which of the following features describe trigeminal neuralgia?**

A   Dull ache

B   Electric shock-like

C   Activated by touching a trigger zone

D   Usually prevents patients' sleeping

E   Lasts for hours

3.4   BDE

Primary herpetic gingivostomatitis is a viral infection. Therefore it is not treated with antibiotics or anti-fungals. Aciclovir can be used in severe cases and when there is widespread infection, but it needs to be given early. In milder cases bed rest, analgesics and fluids are usually sufficient

3.5   ACD

In secondary Sjögren's syndrome, either xerostomia (dry mouth) or xerophthalmia (dry eyes) occurs in association with an autoimmune connective tissue disorder. Patients do not lose their sense of smell (anosmia) or have a higher incidence of oral SCC.

3.6   BC

Trigeminal neuralgia is an intense, excruciating, paroxysmal pain, often described as a shooting or electric shock-like pain. It lasts seconds and usually occurs when a trigger zone is touched. It does not usually keep patients awake at night.

3.7 **Which of the following can be used to treat trigeminal neuralgia?**

A   Jaw exercises in retruded position

B   Carbamazepine

C   Baclofen

D   Phenytoin

E   Flumazenil

3.8 **Which of the following drugs has gingival hyperplasia as a side effect?**

A   Phenytoin

B   Carbamazepine

C   Nifedipine

D   Cisplatin

E   Ciclosporin

3.9 **Which of the following conditions are strongly associated with human immunodeficiency virus (HIV) infection?**

A   Kaposi's carcinoma

B   Hairy leukoplakia

C   Candidiasis

D   Lichen planus

E   Necrotising ulcerative gingivitis

3.7 BCD

Retruded jaw exercises are helpful in the management of temporomandibular joint dysfunction. Flumazenil is a benzodiazepine antagonist used for the reversal of the central sedative effects of benzodiazepines. Carbamazepine, baclofen and phenytoin may all be used for the treatment of trigeminal neuralgia.

3.8 ACE

Gingival hyperplasia is a common side effect of calcium-channel blockers such as nifedipine and diltiazem. It also occurs with phenytoin and ciclosporin.

3.9 BCE

Kaposi's sarcoma is commonly associated with HIV infection. Hairy leukoplakia is strongly associated with HIV; non-HIV cases do occur but usually in immunocompromised patients. Candidal infections are extremely common in HIV-infected patients as is periodontal disease including acute necrotising ulcerative gingivitis.

3.10   Which of the following drugs commonly cause lichenoid reactions?

A   Gold

B   Non-steroidal anti-inflammatory drugs (NSAIDs)

C β-Blockers

D   Carbamazepine

E   Oral hypoglycaemics

3.11   Which of the following are types of lichen planus?

A   Reticular

B   Erosive

C   Pseudomembranous

D   Bullous

E   Hyperplastic

3.12   Which of the following are treatments options for lichen planus?

A   No treatment

B   Fluconazole

C   Triamcinolone acetonide

D   Azathioprine

E   Pilocarpine

3.10 ABCE

Many drugs have been found to cause lichenoid reactions including anti-malarials, NSAIDs, gold, some tricyclic antidepressants, oral hypoglycaemics, methyldopa, penicillamine and β-blockers.

3.11 ABD

Six types of lichen planus have been described: reticular, papular, plaque-like, atrophic (desquamative gingivitis), erosive/ulcerative and bullous. Pseudomembranous and hyperplastic are types of candidiasis.

3.12 ACD

Treatment is not always required for lichen planus, and depends on the severity. Active treatment ranges from topical to systemic corticosteroids. In severe cases immunosuppressants, eg azathioprine and ciclosporin, may be necessary. Fluconazole is an anti-fungal used for the treatment of candidiasis. Pilocarpine is a parasympathomimetic used in the treatment of dry mouth.

3.13 **Which of the following conditions are associated with bullous lesions?**

A   Epidermolysis bullosa

B   Linear Ig A disease

C   Erythema multiforme

D   Pemphigus

E   Bulimia

3.14 **Which of the following statements are true?**

A   Lichen planus is characterised by mononuclear inflammatory infiltrate in the lamina propria

B   The rate of malignant transformation with lichen planus is in the order of 10%

C   Patients with systemic lupus erythematosus (SLE) may present with a malar rash

D   Pemphigus is more common in children

E   Behçet's syndrome may present with conjunctivitis and uveitis

3.15 **Which of the following are true regarding Sjögren's syndrome?**

A   It is more common in females

B   Primary Sjögren's may be associated with rheumatoid arthritis

C   Autoantibodies against ribonucleotide are found: SS-A or Ro and SS-B or La

D   May lead to B-cell lymphoma (MALTOMA)

E   Tricyclic antidepressants may be helpful

3.13 ABD

Epidermolysis bullosa and pemphigus may present with bullous lesions, as may linear IgA disease. Bulimia presents with tooth erosion, and erythema multiforme presents with ulcers and blood-stained, crusted lips.

3.14 ACE

The rate of malignant transformation with lichen planus is in the order of 1%. Pemphigus is found mainly in middle-aged and older patients. SLE patients present with the classic malar 'butterfly' rash.

3.15 ACD

Secondary Sjögren's syndrome comprises dry eyes or dry mouth together with a connective tissue or autoimmune disease – not primary Sjögren's syndrome. Dry mouth is a side effect of tricyclic antidepressants.

3.16 Regarding aphthous ulcers:

A They are more common in males

B The herpetiform-type are more common in males

C Haematinic deficiencies are detected in approximately 50% of cases

D They can be associated with cessation of smoking

E They are often helped by the used of antidepressants

3.17 Which of the following lesions/conditions are caused by viruses?

A Koplik's spots

B Herpetiform ulcers

C Herpes labialis

D Ramsay–Hunt syndrome

E Lyme disease

3.18 Patients with which of the following conditions are more likely to get oral candidal infections than those without?

A Patients undergoing chemotherapy

B Sjögren's syndrome

C Diabetes mellitus

D Anaemia

E Malnourishment

3.16 D

Aphthous ulcers are slightly commoner in females than males. Haematinic deficiencies are detected in up to 20% of patients, and the ulcers can sometimes be associated with smoking cessation. The main treatment after correction of haematinic deficiencies is topical corticosteroids.

3.17 ACD

Koplik's spots are seen in the buccal mucosa in patients with measles, which is an infection caused by paramyxovirus. Herpes labialis is caused by the herpes simplex virus and Ramsay–Hunt syndrome is due to herpes zoster of the geniculate ganglion. Herpetiform ulcers are a type of aphthous ulcer and are not caused by a virus. Lyme disease is caused by *Borrelia burgdorferi*, a spirochaetal bacterium, and is spread via ticks.

3.18 ABCDE

Candidal infections are commoner in patients with other underlying disease processes. Hence patients with anaemia, diabetes mellitus and those who are malnourished or undergoing chemotherapy are more at risk of candidal infections. Patients with Sjögren's syndrome suffer from dry mouth, which puts them at greater risk of candidal infections.

3.19 Which of the following conditions can be associated with oral mucosal disease?

A Crohn's disease

B Irritable bowel syndrome (IBS)

C Ulcerative colitis

D Peutz–Jeghers syndrome

E Bowen's disease

3.20 Which of the following are treatments for dry mouth?

A Pilocarpine

B Salivary substitutes based on carboxymethylcellulose

C Mucin-based salivary substitutes

D Atropine

E Hyoscine

3.21 Angular cheilitis can be:

A Caused by candidal infection of the commissures

B Caused by *Staphylococcus aureus* infection of the commissures

C Caused by an increase in occlusal vertical dimension in patients wearing dentures

D Treated with aciclovir cream

E Treated with miconazole cream

3.19 ACD

Bowen's disease is carcinoma-in-situ of the skin. Crohn's disease may affect any part of the gastrointestinal tract and hence the oral cavity may be involved. Lesions seen are cobblestoning of the buccal mucosa, glossitis, mucosal tags and swelling of the lips. In Peutz–Jeghers syndrome pigmented macules are seen around the peri-oral region. In ulcerative colitis, aphthous ulcers may be seen possibly due to the malabsorption which accompanies the condition. IBS is not usually associated with oral lesions.

3.20 ABC

Pilocarpine stimulates muscarinic receptors in the salivary glands and hence increases the production of saliva. It is used for patients who have some residual salivary gland function following radiotherapy. Artificial saliva may be used for symptomatic relief of dry mouth and can be based on carboxymethylcellulose or mucin. Atropine and hyoscine are anti-muscarinic drugs that dry up secretions.

3.21 ABE

Angular cheilitis is a combined staphylococcal and fungal infection that occurs at the angles of the mouth. It has been previously attributed to a decreased occlusal vertical dimension in denture wearers, but increasing the vertical dimension alone will not treat the infection. Treatment can involve fusidic acid cream and an antifungal, eg miconazole. Aciclovir is an anti-viral medication and hence not indicated for angular cheilitis.

3.22 **Although the aetiology of recurrent aphthous ulceration is unknown, which of the following are thought to be associated with aphthous ulceration?**

    A   Smoking

    B   Haematinic deficiencies

    C   Stress

    D   Family history

    E   HIV

3.23 **Which of the following oral lesions are known to be related to candidal infections?**

    A   Antibiotic sore mouth

    B   Denture stomatitis

    C   Median rhomboid glossitis

    D   Geographical tongue (erythema migrans)

    E   Hairy leukoplakia

3.24 **Dry mouth may be caused by:**

    A   Hyperbaric oxygen treatment of osteoradionecrosis

    B   Sjögren's syndrome

    C   Sarcoidosis

    D   Bell's palsy

    E   Parkinson's disease

3.22 BCDE

The cause of recurrent aphthous ulceration is unknown, but several associations have been made. Stress, haematinic deficiencies and a family history all predispose a patient to getting aphthae. The ulcers also occur in HIV infections, being more severe in the more immunocompromised cases. Smoking is not associated with aphthae, in fact patients who do not smoke or who have recently stopped smoking are more likely to suffer from aphthae.

3.23 ABC

Antibiotic sore mouth and denture stomatitis are caused by candidal infection. Previously median rhomboid glossitis was thought to be a developmental condition, but it is now thought to be due to chronic atrophic candidal infection on the tongue. The cause of geographic tongue is unknown. Hairy leukoplakia occurs in HIV-infected patients and immunocompromised individuals. The lesion may be secondarily infected with *Candida*, but it is not the cause of the lesion.

3.24 BC

Bell's palsy and Parkinson's disease are commonly associated with hypersalivation (ptyalism). Hyperbaric oxygen treatment does not cause a dry mouth although the patients may have a dry mouth following the radiotherapy. Both Sjögren's syndrome and sarcoidosis may cause a dry mouth.

3.25 **Regarding oral cancer:**

A   It accounts for approximately 10% of cancers in the UK

B   It is commoner in men

C   Smoking and heavy alcohol intake are synergistic risk factors

D   Chewed tobacco (betel nut) is safer than smoked tobacco

E   It may arise in white patches

3.26 **Which of the following are potentially malignant oral lesions?**

A   Oral submucosal fibrosis

B   Speckled leukoplakia

C   Actinic cheilitis

D   Erythema migrans

E   Erythema multiforme

3.27 **Regarding mucous membrane pemphigoid:**

A   It is commoner in men

B   The onset is in the third to fourth decade

C   It is characterised by deposits of immunoglobulins and complement components in the basement membrane

D   It is characterised by loss of intercellular adherence of supra-basal spinous cells

E   Ocular involvement may lead to blindness

3.25 BCE ·

Oral cancer accounts for approximately 2% of cancers in the UK, and traditionally it was a disease of older men. However, the incidence is increasing in younger patients and women. Smoking and alcohol consumption are risk factors and are thought to act synergistically. Chewing betel nut is also a risk factor and important in the Indian subcontinent where it is commonly practised. White patches in the mouth have a potential for malignant change.

3.26 ABC

Various potentially malignant conditions occur in the oral cavity. The lesion with the highest rate of malignant transformation is erythroplasia. Speckled leukoplakia and leukoplakia also have the potential to turn malignant. Oral submucous fibrosis, lichen planus, actinic cheilitis, chronic hyperplastic candidosis and lupus erythematosus are all potentially malignant lesions.

3.27 CE

Loss of intercellular adherence of supra-basal spinous cells is characteristic of pemphigus vulgaris; in pemphigoid the split occurs at the level of the basement membrane. Mucous membrane pemphigoid is twice as common in women and usually affects people in their fifth to sixth decades. One complication of the disease is ocular involvement, which may lead to scarring and blindness.

3.28 Desquamative gingivitis is seen in which of the following conditions?

A   Lichen planus

B   Pemphigus vulgaris

C   Erythema multiforme

D   Erythema migrans

E   Mucous membrane pemphigoid

3.29 Regarding Bell's palsy:

A   It is an upper motor neurone lesion

B   It causes a unilateral paralysis of all the muscles of facial expression

C   It is thought to be due to compression of the facial nerve in the pterygomaxillary fissure

D   Loss of taste may also be associated

E   It is usually treated with low-dose steroids

3.30 Regarding herpes infections of the trigeminal area:

A   Reactivation of the herpes simplex virus usually causes cold sores on the lips

B   Herpetic whitlows can be caught only from patients with primary herpes infections

C   Post-herpetic neuralgia follows a herpes simplex infection

D   Post-herpetic neuralgia usually responds well to treatment with carbamazepine

E   Post-herpetic neuralgia usually occurs in young patients

3.28 ABE

In desquamative gingivitis, the gingivae are red, inflamed and atrophic. It occurs in lichen planus, pemphigus vulgaris and mucous membrane pemphigoid.

3.29 BD

Bell's palsy is a lower motor neurone lesion of the facial nerve, and as such it causes unilateral paralysis of all the muscles of facial expression. Upper motor neurone lesions affecting the facial nerve do not cause paralysis of the forehead as there is some cross-over in innervation. The palsy is thought to be due to compression of the facial nerve in the stylomastoid canal. Loss of taste occurs due to the chorda tympani being affected. Treatment is usually with high-dose steroids initially, which are then tailed off.

3.30 A

Reactivation of the herpes simplex virus does cause herpes labialis, which takes the form of cold sores on the lips. Herpetic whitlows can be caught from patients with primary or secondary herpetic infections. Post-herpetic neuralgia follows herpes zoster infection, and usually occurs in older people. The response to carbamazepine is often poor.

4

Oral
Pathology

4.1 Which of the following are microscopic features of epithelial dysplasia?

A Atypical mitosis

B Hyperkeratinisation

C Loss of cellular polarity

D Altered nuclear/cytoplasmic ratio

E Loss or reduction of intercellular adherence

4.2 Which of the following microscopic features are suggestive of the white lesion of lichen planus?

A Saw tooth rete ridges

B Hypokeratosis

C Dense band of macrophages below the basement membrane

D Basal cell liquefaction

E Acantholysis

4.3 Carcinoma of the lip:

A Is commoner in the upper lip

B Is often caused by chewing betel nut/paan

C Has a worse prognosis than intra-oral carcinoma

D Is principally caused by alcohol consumption

E Often occurs in patients with submucous fibrosis

4.1   ACDE

Dysplasia is a term used to describe histological abnormalities seen in both premalignant and malignant cells. Abnormal features include: abnormal mitoses and increased number of mitoses; loss of polarity; drop-shaped rete ridges; abnormal intercellular adherence; and abnormal nuclear/cytoplasmic ratio. Abnormal keratinisation occurs in cells situated more basally than in the layers in which cells normally keratinise. Hyperkeratinisation is not a feature of dysplasia.

4.2   AD

The typical histological features of lichen planus include saw tooth rete ridges, hyperkeratosis or parakeratosis, a dense band of lymphocytes below the basement membrane and basal cell liquefaction.

4.3   All statements are false

Carcinoma of the lip is commoner on the lower lip. It is often identified early because it is visible and hence has a better prognosis than intra-oral carcinoma. The main risk factor for carcinoma of the lip is exposure to sunlight, and it is not affected by alcohol consumption or betel nut chewing in the same way as intra-oral carcinoma. Intra-oral carcinoma commonly occurs in patients with submucous fibrosis.

4.4   In anhidrotic ectodermal dysplasia:

A   There are often supernumerary teeth

B   Hair is usually scanty

C   A sex-linked recessive trait is usually the cause

D   Anhidrosis refers to the type of hair present

E   Teeth are often peg shaped

4.5   Delayed eruption of teeth is a feature of which of the following conditions?

A   Cleidocranial dysostosis

B   Osteogenesis imperfecta

C   Rickets

D   Cherubism

E   Scurvy

4.6   Regarding dental fluorosis:

A   It affects deciduous teeth and permanent teeth equally

B   It causes white or brownish mottling of teeth

C   Mottled teeth are less susceptible to caries than teeth not exposed to fluoride

D   It occurs in areas when fluoride in the drinking water exceeds 1 ppm

E   It occurs in areas when fluoride in the drinking water exceeds 2 ppm

4.4 BCE

Anhidrotic ectodermal dysplasia is usually a sex-linked recessive trait that results in hypodontia, hypotrichosis (scanty and wispy hair) and anhidrosis (inability to sweat). Any teeth present are often peg shaped or conical.

4.5 ACD

Delayed eruption of teeth usually occurs in cleidocranial dysostosis and rickets. In cherubism eruption may be delayed due to displacement by the giant cell lesions.

4.6 BCE

Excess fluoride ingestion causes dental fluorosis. Fluoride is usually present in drinking water and effects are seen when it exceeds 2 ppm. Mottling of the teeth occurs and appears as white or brown areas on the teeth with varying degrees of pitting. Permanent teeth are usually affected – it rarely affects deciduous teeth.

4.7   Regarding dental caries:

A   Lactobacilli are the bacteria that are the main cause of dental caries

B   Cariogenic bacteria produce acid

C   Glucose is more cariogenic than sucrose

D   Fructose is less cariogenic than sucrose

E   Sugar alcohols (polyols) are cariogenic

4.8   Acute osteomyelitis:

A   Affects the maxilla more commonly than the mandible

B   Always causes paraesthesia in relation to the inferior dental nerve

C   Will not be apparent on radiographs until about 10 days

D   Usually causes sharp, shooting pain

E   May cause associated teeth to loosen

4.9   Regarding actinomycosis:

A   It is a suppurative infection caused by a coccal bacterium, usually *Actinomyces israelii*

B   It is more common in women than men

C   It usually affects middle-aged people

D   Multiple discharging sinuses are seen, and the pus contains 'sulphur granules' (bacterial colonies)

E   It is treated with metronidazole

4.7   BD

Viridans streptococci are the most cariogenic bacteria and not lactobacilli, which tend to appear in bacterial plaque after caries has developed. All cariogenic bacteria produce acid. The most cariogenic sugar is sucrose – both glucose and fructose are less cariogenic than sucrose. Sugar alcohols are non-cariogenic and so are used in 'sugar-free' foods.

4.8   CE

Acute osteomyelitis commonly affects the mandible. Osteomyelitis of the maxilla is rare although it may occur in infants. Acute osteomyelitis is associated with severe, deep-seated, throbbing pain, the associated teeth become tender and loose, and pus may exude from the socket. Alteration in sensation in relation to the inferior dental nerve may occur, but not in all cases.

Radiographic changes are not visible initially, only becoming apparent after about 10 days, when loss of trabeculae and areas of bone destruction are evident.

4.9   CD

Actinomycosis is a suppurative infection that is usually caused by *Actinomyces israelii*, a filamentous bacterium. It most commonly tends to affect men aged about 30–60 years. Multiple discharging sinuses are seen, and the pus contains granules known as 'sulphur granules', which are colonies of *Actinomyces* species. Treatment involves drainage of the pus along with penicillin or tetracycline.

4.10 Regarding radicular cysts:

A   The cyst capsule often contains cholesterol crystals

B   The cyst fluid often shimmers due to the keratin contained within

C   The cyst lining is formed of stratified squamous epithelium

D   Rushton's bodies in the cyst wall indicate that the cyst is actively growing

E   Radicular cysts are always associated with a non-vital pulp

4.11 Keratocysts:

A   Are always multilocular

B   Are commoner in the mandible than the maxilla

C   Grow along the bone rather than expanding the jaw

D   Are always associated with a missing tooth

E   Commonly recur

4.12 Patients with Gorlin–Goltz syndrome (or basal cell carcinoma/jaw cyst syndrome) have:

A   Multiple radicular cysts

B   Frontal and parietal bossing

C   Multiple basal cell carcinomas of the skin

D   Supernumerary teeth

E   Skeletal abnormalities such as bifid ribs and vertebral abnormalities

4.10 ACE

Radicular cysts are formed following infection or inflammation of the pulp and are associated with non-vital roots. The cyst lining is formed of stratified squamous epithelium, which contains hyaline or Rushton's bodies, which indicate the odontogenic origin of the cyst. The cyst capsule contains cholesterol crystals and the cholesterol in the cyst fluid gives it a shimmering appearance.

4.11 BCE

Keratocysts are often unilocular when small and become multilocular as they enlarge. They are thought to be formed from the remnants of the dental lamina and so are not always associated with a missing tooth. They are commoner in the mandible than the maxilla. They commonly recur due to the difficulty of removing all of the friable lining.

4.12 BCE

The features of Gorlin–Goltz syndrome are multiple keratocysts, multiple basal cell carcinomas, intra-cranial abnormalities such as calcification of the falx cerebri, and frontal bossing and other skeletal abnormalities including bifid ribs.

4.13 In syphilis:

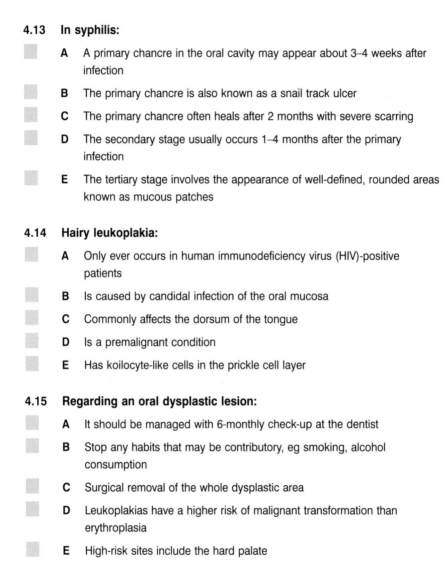

A   A primary chancre in the oral cavity may appear about 3–4 weeks after infection

B   The primary chancre is also known as a snail track ulcer

C   The primary chancre often heals after 2 months with severe scarring

D   The secondary stage usually occurs 1–4 months after the primary infection

E   The tertiary stage involves the appearance of well-defined, rounded areas known as mucous patches

4.14 Hairy leukoplakia:

A   Only ever occurs in human immunodeficiency virus (HIV)-positive patients

B   Is caused by candidal infection of the oral mucosa

C   Commonly affects the dorsum of the tongue

D   Is a premalignant condition

E   Has koilocyte-like cells in the prickle cell layer

4.15 Regarding an oral dysplastic lesion:

A   It should be managed with 6-monthly check-up at the dentist

B   Stop any habits that may be contributory, eg smoking, alcohol consumption

C   Surgical removal of the whole dysplastic area

D   Leukoplakias have a higher risk of malignant transformation than erythroplasia

E   High-risk sites include the hard palate

4.13   AD

An oral chancre appears in primary syphilis about 3–4 weeks after infection. It often heals without scarring after a couple of months. In secondary syphilis the oral lesions consist of ulcers that are covered with a greyish slough known as snail track ulcers. When ulcers join together, larger areas are involved and these are known as mucous patches. The lesion in tertiary syphilis is the gumma.

4.14   E

Hairy leukoplakia occurs most commonly in homosexual men infected with HIV. It also occurs in immunodeficient patients although it is not as common. It is often secondarily infected with *Candida*, and occurs most commonly on the lateral borders of the tongue. It is not a premalignant condition. Histologically there is hyperkeratosis or parakeratosis. In the prickle cell layer are vacuolated and ballooned cells with dark nuclei surrounded by a clear halo – koilocyte-like cells.

4.15   B

Dysplastic lesions should be reviewed 3 months after elimination of risk factors and regularly thereafter. Surgical excision of the lesion may be indicated if the lesion persists, depending on the degree of dysplasia, and site and extent of the lesion. Erythroplasia (erythroplakia) and non-homogeneous leukoplakias have a much higher risk of malignant transformation than homogeneous leukoplakias. The high-risk sites include the ventrolateral surfaces of the tongue, floor of the mouth and soft palate/fauces.

4.16   Salivary calculi:

   A   Commonly cause dry mouth

   B   Occur most commonly in the sublingual gland

   C   Occur most commonly in the parotid gland

   D   Are always visible on radiographs

   E   May be asymptomatic

4.17   With respect to salivary gland tumours:

   A   About 75% of all salivary gland tumours occur in the parotid gland

   B   About 10% of all salivary gland tumours occur in the minor salivary glands

   C   A tumour in the parotid gland is more likely to be malignant than a tumour in the minor salivary glands

   D   Most tumours in the sublingual salivary gland are benign

   E   The commonest salivary gland tumour is a adenoid cystic carcinoma

4.18   With respect to salivary gland tumours:

   A   Pleomorphic adenomas usually undergo malignant change

   B   Pleomorphic adenomas may contain fibrous, myxoid and elastic tissue

   C   Mucoepidermoid carcinomas have a characteristic 'Swiss cheese' pattern

   D   Acinic cell carcinomas commonly spread along nerve sheaths

   E   Adenoid cystic carcinomas have a poor prognosis

4.16 E

Salivary calculi occur most commonly in the submandibular gland and may be asymptomatic. They are not always visible on radiographs and do not cause a dry mouth.

4.17 AB

About three-quarters of all salivary gland tumours occur in the parotid gland, and about a tenth occur in the minor salivary glands. A tumour in a minor gland is more likely to be malignant as about a third are malignant, whereas in the parotid gland only about 15% are malignant. However, a tumour in the sublingual gland is most likely to be malignant as over 80% of tumours in this site are malignant. The commonest salivary gland tumour is the pleomorphic adenoma.

4.18 BE

Only about 2–4% of pleomorphic adenomas undergo malignant change. They may contain a wide variety of tissue types including fibrous, myxoid and elastic. The characteristic 'Swiss cheese' appearance and spread along nerve sheaths is seen in adenoid cystic carcinomas. Adenoid cystic carcinomas grow slowly, metastasise late, and have a poor prognosis.

4.19 Which of the following investigations are appropriate for the lesions?

A   Incisional biopsy for a suspected squamous cell carcinoma

B   Incisional biopsy for a suspected haemangioma

C   Excisional biopsy for a suspected fibroepithelial polyp

D   Excisional biopsy for a white patch of unknown origin

E   Incisional biopsy for a mucous extravasation cyst

4.20 Regarding ameloblastoma:

A   It usually presents between the ages of 15 and 20 years

B   It is the commonest odontogenic neoplasm

C   It presents as a monolocular cyst on radiographs

D   It is common in the posterior mandible

E   Follicular ameloblastoma is the commonest type

4.21 With respect to fibrous dysplasia:

A   It is commoner in females

B   It typically affects the maxilla

C   It is painful

D   Histologically there is irregular resorption and deposition of bone

E   Commonly occurs in the fourth decade

4.19 AC

Incisional biopsies should be done on squamous cell carcinomas and white patches of unknown origin. An excisional biopsy is appropriate for a fibroepithelial polyp and a mucous extravasation cyst. Biopsy should not be attempted on a suspected haemangioma.

4.20 BDE

Ameloblastoma usually presents between the ages of 30 and 50 years, and it presents as a multilocular cyst. The other types of ameloblastoma are: plexiform, acanthomatous, basal cell and granular cell. Unicystic ameloblastomas are considered as a distinct entity to the solid variants of ameloblastoma.

4.21 AB

In fibrous dysplasia normal bone is replaced by fibrous tissue. It usually affects the maxilla and people below the age of 20. It is not often painful. Irregular resorption and deposition of bone is seen in Paget's disease.

4.22 With respect to osteosarcoma:

A   It is a complication of Paget's disease

B   It is commoner in the maxilla

C   Paraesthesia may be the presenting feature

D   It is commoner in males

E   It is most commonly seen in children

4.23 Regarding hyperparathyroidism:

A   It is characterised by raised plasma calcium levels

B   It presents with giant cell lesions

C   Jaw lesions are commonly present

D   Patients may present with enlargement of the skull

E   It is most commonly secondary to chronic renal failure (CRF)

4.24 Which of the following are true of cherubism?

A   It is a rare genetic defect of osteoclastic activity

B   It is commoner in males

C   The middle third of the face is usually hypoplastic

D   Presents with lesions also known as Brown's tumours

E   Regression of the disease occurs

4.22 ACD

Osteosarcoma is rare and more common in the mandible. It is most commonly seen between the ages of 30 and 40 years and in males. It occurs as a complication of Paget's disease, although it is not common.

4.23 ABE

Skull enlargement occurs with Paget's disease. Osteolytic lesions in bone are more commonly the result of secondary hyperparathyroidism (eg CRF) than primary (hyperplasia or adenoma of parathyroids).

4.24 ABE

Cherubism is inherited as an autosomal dominant trait. It presents with expansion of the maxilla. Brown tumours are seen secondary to hyperparathyroidism.

4.25 **Which of the following are potentially malignant oral lesions/ conditions?**

A Speckled leukoplakia

B Tertiary syphilis

C Paterson–Kelly syndrome

D Chronic candidiasis

E Medium rhomboid glossitis

4.26 **Regarding Warthin's tumour (adenolymphoma):**

A It is commoner in males

B Tall columnar eosinophilic cells covering lymphoid tissue is the characteristic histological appearance

C It is the commonest type of salivary tumour

D Average age of presentation is 40 years

E 10% are bilateral

4.27 **Which of the following features would raise suspicion of a malignant salivary tumour?**

A Facial nerve palsy

B Soft rubbery consistency

C Sudden increase in size

D Lesion is in a minor salivary gland rather than in the parotid

E Skin ulceration

4.25 ABCD

Various potentially malignant conditions occur in the oral cavity including erythroplasia, dysplastic and speckled leuokplakia, oral submucous fibrosis, tertiary syphilis, chronic candidiasis and lichen planus. There is also high incidence of oral and oesophageal cancer in Paterson-Kelly syndrome. Median rhomboid glossitis is not a potentially malignant lesion.

4.26 ABE

The male to female ratio of occurrence of Warthin's tumour is 7:1. It is a benign tumour, making up 7–8% of salivary tumours. The average age of presentation is 70 years; 40 years is the average age for presentation of pleomorphic adenomas.

4.27 ACDE

A mass of hard consistency is more likely to be malignant. Sudden increase in size of a salivary mass, even if it has been present for many years, should alert the clinician to a risk of malignant mass. Pain, nerve involvement and nodal metastases are also signs of malignant growth.

4.28 Which of the following are true of oral submucous fibrosis:

A   It is associated with smoking

B   It is at risk of malignant transformation

C   It is managed by topical corticosteroids

D   It characteristically affects the buccal mucosa

E   It may present with trismus

4.29 Regarding odontomes:

A   They are hamartomas

B   They usually present around the age of 30 years

C   They can undergo malignant transformation

D   They most commonly present in the anterior maxilla

E   The lesion is composed of cementum embedded in fibrous tissue and a surrounding capsule

4.30 Which of the following statements are true?

A   Ameloblastic fibromas usually present around the age of 50 years

B   Ghost and ameloblastic cells are characteristically seen in ameloblastic fibromas

C   Calcifying epithelial odontogenic tumour is also known as Pindborg's tumour

D   Calcifying epithelial odontogenic tumours are locally invasive

E   Adenomatoid odontogenic tumours most commonly present in the anterior maxilla

4.28 BDE

Oral submucous fibrosis is associated with betel quid chewing (smokeless tobacco). Intra-lesional injections of steroids have been tried, but the benefit is limited. The risk of malignant transformation is reported to be around 5–8%.

4.29 AD

Odontomes usually present between the ages of 10 and 20 years, and are benign lesions. They most commonly present in the anterior maxilla and posterior mandible. The lesion is composed of pulp, dentine, enamel and cementum.

4.30 CDE

Ameloblastic fibromas usually present in children or young adults. Ghost and ameloblastic cells are seen in calcifying odontogenic cysts.

5

Oral
Surgery

5.1 **According to the National Institute for Health and Clinical Excellence (NICE) guidelines, which of the following are indications for the removal of a lower third molar tooth?**

A   Crowding of lower anterior teeth

B   Single episode of mild pericoronitis

C   A contralateral tooth requiring removal under general anaesthetic

D   Treatment of facial pain

E   Mesioangular impaction

5.2 **Which of the following statements regarding cranial nerves are true?**

A   The abducent nerve supplies the superior oblique muscle

B   The motor supply to the muscles of mastication comes from the facial nerve

C   Sensation and taste to the posterior third of the tongue are supplied by the hypoglossal nerve

D   The trigeminal nerve is motor to the muscles of mastication

E   The lower face has bilateral facial nerve innervation

5.3 **Temporal arteritis:**

A   May cause blindness

B   Is commoner in women

C   Is treated with non-steroidal anti-inflammatory drugs (NSAIDs)

D   Results in a lowered erythrocyte sedimentation rate (ESR)

E   Causes pain in the face

5.1 All statements are false

The NICE guidelines for the removal of wisdom teeth state that none of the above are indications for removal of lower third molars. A single episode of pericoronitis could be an indication – provided that it is a severe episode.

5.2 D

The abducent nerve supplies the lateral rectus muscle of the eye; the superior oblique muscle is supplied by the trochlear nerve. The motor supply to the muscles of mastication comes from the trigeminal nerve whereas the facial nerve is motor to the muscles of facial expression. The hypoglossal nerve is motor to all the muscles of the tongue (except palatoglossus), and the glossopharyngeal nerve supplies the sensory supply to the posterior third of the tongue. The lower face has unilateral facial nerve innervation, whereas the upper face is bilaterally innervated.

5.3 ABE

Temporal arteritis or giant cell arteritis may cause blindness. It is commoner in women and results in a raised ESR, causes facial pain and is usually treated with steroids.

5.4   Which of the following muscles open(s) the mouth?

A   Masseter muscle

B   Temporalis muscle

C   Lateral pterygoid muscle

D   Digastric muscle

E   Medial pterygoid muscle

5.5   Deviation of the mandible on opening could be due to:

A   A unilateral anteriorly displaced disc

B   Ankylosis of one condyle

C   An occlusal interference between the retruded contact position (RCP) and intercuspal position (ICP)

D   Internal derangement of the temporomandibular joint (TMJ)

E   A fractured condyle

5.6   Cluster headache:

A   Is more common in males

B   Usually affects patients > 50 years of age

C   May be associated with nasal congestion, watering of the eyes and facial flushing

D   Can only be treated with ergotamine

E   Is usually diagnosed with a computed tomography (CT) or magnetic resonance imaging (MRI) scan

5.4 CD

The masseter and medial pterygoid muscles close the mouth, as do the anterior fibres of the temporalis muscle. The lateral pterygoid and digastric muscles both open the mouth.

5.5 ABDE

Any interference with normal condylar movement may cause the mandible to deviate on opening. If the interference is on one side then the mandible usually deviates towards that side on opening as the condyle is unable to translate forward, whilst the condyle on the normal side translates forward. Occlusal interferences do not usually interfere with mandibular opening, but with closing.

5.6 AC

Cluster headache (alarm clock headache) is an intense pain centred over the temporal and eye region. There is parasympathetic activity, as the headache is often associated with facial flushing and sweating, lacrimation and rhinorrhoea, as well as ptosis and nasal congestion. It is commoner in males, usually younger than 50 years. Diagnosis is usually made on the basis of the history, although imaging may be done to rule out pathology. Treatment is symptomatic, with 'triptans' which are 5-hydroxytryptamine (5-HT) agonists or ergot alkaloids.

5.7   Glossopharyngeal neuralgia:

A   Is more common that trigeminal neuralgia

B   Is usually described as a dull ache

C   May be felt in the ear on the affected side

D   Affects the postero-lateral side of the tongue

E   Is easily amenable to cryotherapy of the nerve

5.8   Regarding the maxillary sinus:

A   It is not present at birth

B   In adults it is pyramidal in shape with the base lying medially

C   It drains via the ostium into the inferior meatus of the nose

D   It is lined by pseudostratified ciliated columnar epithelium

E   It is the largest of the paranasal sinuses

5.9   Osteoradionecrosis (or irradiation osteomyelitis):

A   Is a suppurative type of osteomyelitis

B   Affects the maxilla more commonly than the mandible

C   Occurs due to a reduction in vascularity secondary to endarteritis obliterans

D   Can occur following hyperbaric oxygen treatment for squamous cell carcinoma

E   Is the same as focal sclerosing osteomyelitis

5.7 CD

Glossopharyngeal neuralgia is rare, but has the same intensity as paroxysmal trigeminal neuralgia. It may be felt in the ear as well as on the posterior third of the tongue. As the glossopharyngeal nerve is difficult to access, the condition is not amenable to cryotherapy.

5.8 BDE

The maxillary sinus is the first of the paranasal sinuses to develop and is approximately 1 cm in diameter at birth. It is pyramidal in shape with its base lying medially, forming the lateral wall of the nose. It drains via the ostium into the middle meatus of the nose.

5.9 C

Osteoradionecrosis occurs following radiotherapy to the jaws. It occurs as the bone becomes less vascular and hypocellular after the radiation treatment. It usually affects the mandible more than the maxilla. It is not caused by treatment with hyperbaric oxygen, but hyperbaric oxygen is often used to treat it. It is not a suppurating type of osteomyelitis. Focal sclerosing osteomyelitis is a rare condition thought to be due to a reaction to a low-grade infection that usually affects children and young adults. It is a different entity from osteoradionecrosis.

5.10 In the TMN classification system:

A   A 1.5 cm tumour on the lateral border of the tongue with no palpable neck nodes would be classified as stage 1

B   Stages are based solely on histopathological grades

C   The N classification relates only to lymph nodes on the ipsilateral side to the tumour

D   Nx means that the patient has undergone a previous neck dissection

E   M1 means distant metastasis

5.11 The submandibular gland:

A   Is the largest of the salivary glands

B   Empties via Stensen's duct

C   Has a duct that is closely related to the lingual nerve

D   Is the gland most commonly affected by salivary gland calculi

E   Is a mixed salivary gland

5.12 Dry mouth:

A   Can be caused by radiation therapy

B   Can occur in diabetes mellitus

C   Can occur with anxiety

D   Occurs when the salivary flow rate falls below the normal of 1 ml/min

E   Can result in an increase in root caries

5.10   AE

The TMN (*T*umour, *N*ode, *M*etastasis) is a clinical and pathological classification system used in cancer cases. The classification is shown below.

Primary tumour	T	
	Tx	Primary tumour cannot be assessed
	T0	No evidence of primary tumour
	Tis	Carcinoma in situ
	T1	Tumour < 2 cm
	T2	Tumour 2–4 cm
	T3	Tumour > 4 cm
	T4	Tumour invades adjacent structures
Lymph nodes	N	
	Nx	Regional nodes cannot be assessed
	N0	No regional node metastasis
	N1	Metastasis in a single ipsilateral lymph node < 3 cm
	N2	Metastasis in: a single ipsilateral lymph node 3–6 cm
		in multiple ipsilateral nodes < 6 cm
		bilateral or contralateral nodes < 6 cm
	N3	Metastasis in node > 6 cm
Distant metastasis	M	
	Mx	Metastasis cannot be assessed
	M0	No distant metastasis
	M1	Distant metastasis

The stage of disease can be determined from the TNM classification as shown in the following table.

Stage	T level	N level	M level
0	Tis	N0	M0
I	T1	N0	M0
II	T2	N0	M0
III	T3	N0	M0
	T1/2	N1	M0
IV	T4	N0/1	M0
	Any T	N2/3	M0
	Any T	Any N	M1

5.11   CDE

The parotid is the largest salivary gland and it empties via Stensen's duct. The submandibular duct empties via Wharton's duct. The lingual nerve loops underneath Wharton's duct at the posterior aspect of the floor of the mouth. In this position it can easily be damaged during surgery for removing stones. The submandibular salivary gland is a mixed salivary gland and is the gland most commonly affected by salivary calculi.

5.12   ABCE

Diabetes mellitus, irradiation therapy and anxiety can all lead to a dry mouth. It occurs when the salivary flow rate falls below 0.1 ml/min. Dry mouth may result in increased incidence of root caries.

5.13 **Burning mouth syndrome (oral dysaesthesia, glossodynia):**

A   Is more common in females than males

B   Usually affects patients over 50 years of age

C   May occur in patients who are stressed or depressed

D   Is always associated with vitamin B_1 deficiency

E   May respond to treatment with antidepressant drugs

5.14 **The lesion in the figure below is likely to be:**

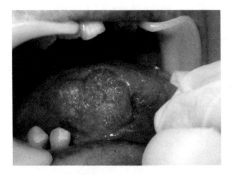

A   Erythema migrans

B   Median rhomboid glossitis

C   Basal cell carcinoma

D   Squamous cell carcinoma

E   Traumatic ulcer

5.15 **The appropriate management of the lesion shown in Q 5.14 may involve:**

A   Incisional biopsy

B   Fine needle aspirate

C   Smear for *Candida*

D   Excisional biopsy

E   Full blood count to rule out haematinic deficiencies as the cause of the oral lesion

5.13   ABCE

Burning mouth syndrome usually affects middle-aged to older women. No physical abnormality is seen. It often occurs in depressed and stressed individuals and as such responds to antidepressive drugs. Haematinic deficiencies may cause burning sensations in the oral cavity, and so should always be investigated in patients complaining of a burning mouth. If found and corrected, the burning sensation should disappear, and as such this is not burning mouth syndrome.

5.14   D

This picture shows an ulcerated area on the lateral border of the tongue. The ulcer is raised with rolled margins. Squamous cell carcinomas of the tongue may present as an ulcer with raised rolled edges. The ulcers are firm to the touch and fixed to surrounding tissue. Erythema migrans (geographical tongue) is seen as smooth red areas on the dorsum of the tongue. Medial rhomboid glossitis is as the name suggests in the mid line of the dorsum of the tongue. Basal cell carcinomas are skin lesions. Traumatic ulcers do not have a raised rolled edge and are often covered in a yellowish slough.

5.15   A

The appropriate management of a suspected oral squamous cell carcinoma is an incisional biopsy.

5.16 Identify the instruments labelled i–v in the figure. Choose from the list of options below.

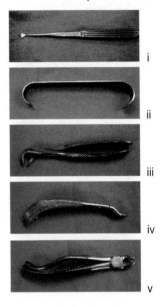

A   i is a Howarth's periosteal elevator

B   ii is a Kilner cheek retractor

C   iii is a pair of lower molar forceps

D   iv is a pair of bayonet forceps

E   v is a pair of upper left molar forceps

5.17 Identify the instruments labelled i–v in the figure. Choose from the list of options below.

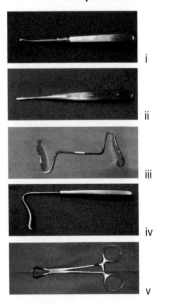

A   i is a left sided Cryer's elevator

B   ii is a Coupland's elevator (chisel)

C   iii is a Lasters' retractor

D   iv is a Bowdler Henry rake retractor

E   v is a pair of Stillies' scissors

5.16   BC

i is a Ward's periosteal elevator, iv is a pair of bayonet forceps used for extracting upper third molar teeth. v is a pair of upper molar forceps for the right not the left, (remember the beak on the forceps goes towards the cheek.)

5.17   AD

ii is a straight Warwick James' elevator. iii is a Ward's buccal retractor and v is a towel clip not a pair of scissors.

5.18 You performed an extraction 3 hours earlier on a fit and healthy patient. The patient has returned to the surgery complaining of bleeding from the extraction site. The appropriate management options are:

A Lie the patient in the chair to calm them down

B Get the patient to bite on a gauze pack

C Pack the socket with Alvogyl®

D Pack the socket with an oxidised cellulose dressing (eg Surgicel®)

E Suture the socket using Prolene sutures

5.19 You are about to extract an upper first permanent molar in a patient who has a large maxillary sinus. What should you warn the patient about prior to the extraction?

A Possibility of an oronasal communication

B Possibility of an oronasal fistula

C Possible infection following the extraction

D Possible pain following the extraction

E Possibility of a nose bleed following the extraction

5.20 You are seeing a patient with an odontogenic infection. Which of the following factors would indicate that this is a severe infection which will require admission to hospital?

A Temperature of 38.5 °C

B Previous episode of pain

C Severe pain

D Tachycardia

E Raised floor of mouth

5.18   BD

It is better to sit the patient upright to reduce the bleeding from the socket. The patient should be made to bite on a gauze pack for at least 5 minutes to assess the effect of continuous pressure on the socket. An appropriate dressing is oxidised cellulose (Surgicel®); Alvogyl® is used for dry sockets. The socket may need to be sutured but Prolene is not the best suture material to use in the mouth because it is a monofilament material and the cut ends are sharp. A braided alternative is better.

5.19   CD

Extraction of an upper first permanent molar in a patient with a large maxillary sinus may result in an oro-antral communication which over time may become epithelialised to form an oro-antral fistula. There is always a possibility of pain and infection after any extraction. There is no need to warn patients of nose bleeds following extractions.

5.20   ADE

Severe odontogenic infections may require hospital admission for treatment. A temperature of 38.5 °C, tachycardia and a raised floor of mouth are all indicators of a severe infection that needs in-patient treatment, so patients with these signs should all be admitted. Pain is not a good indicator of the severity of infection and hence not a good guide to whether a patient needs admission.

5.21 **To which of the following spaces can infection directly spread from a lower wisdom tooth?**

A   Submasseteric space

B   Pterygomaxillary space

C   Submandibular space

D   Cavernous sinus

E   Maxillary sinus

5.22 **This radiograph shows:**

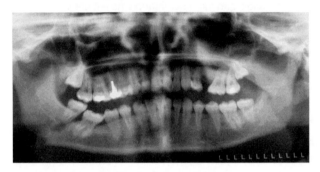

A   a unilateral fractured left condyle

B   a "guardsman" type fracture

C   a bilateral fractured mandible

D   a left mandibular body fracture

E   a left mandibular angle fracture

5.23 **Which method(s) of treatment are appropriate for reduction of a fractured mandibular angle in a dentate patient:**

A   Intramaxillary fixation (IMF) using eyelet wires

B   IMF using arch bars

C   IMF using Gunning splints

D   Mini bone plates

E   IMF using K-wires

5.21 ABC

Infection from a lower wisdom tooth may spread directly to the submasseteric, pterygomaxillary and submandibular spaces. Spread to the cavernous sinus is usually from infections in the middle third of the face. Infection does not spread to the maxillary sinus from lower wisdom teeth.

5.22 CD

This is a dental panoramic radiograph showing a bilateral fractured mandible. One fracture is through the right angle and the other through the left body of the mandible. The condyles appear intact with this view. A "guardsman's" fracture involves bilateral fractured condyles with a symphyseal fracture.

5.23 ABD

IMF is used for fracture reduction, so eyelet wiring and arch bars can be used for mandibular fracture reduction. Previously IMF was left on for 4–6 weeks as a means of fixation until the fracture had healed. Nowadays IMF is used during the operation to achieve the appropriate occlusion but the fracture is fixed with a mini bone plate, and the IMF is released. Gunning splints help achieve IMF in edentulous patients. K-wires are not used for IMF.

5.24 **Which of the following are well-recognised complications of removal of lower wisdom teeth?**

A Paraesthesia of the lingual nerve

B Dry socket

C Anaesthesia of the inferior dental nerve

D Paraesthesia of the inferior dental nerve

E Paralysis of the lingual nerve

5.25 **What are the advantages of marsupialisation of cysts compared with enucleation?**

A Cyst cavity open to inspection

B Whole cyst lining available for histological analysis

C Easier for the patient to look after in terms of oral hygiene

D May be used to prevent damage to vital structures

E Less bone removal

5.26 **Which suture would you use when you want a resorbable suture?**

A Black silk suture 3–0

B Prolene 4–0

C Vicryl 3–0

D Vicryl Rapide 4–0

E Monocryl

5.24 ABCD

Damage to the inferior dental and/or lingual nerves may occur during removal of lower third molars. As these nerves are sensory this may result in anaesthesia or paraesthesia but not paralysis. Dry socket is a common complication of removal of lower molars.

5.25 ADE

Marsupialisation is a technique where the cyst cavity is opened via a window in the lining and this is sutured to the mucosa, so that the cyst cavity communicates with the oral cavity. Enucleation is a technique in which the whole cyst is removed and the cyst cavity closed to the oral cavity. Marsupialisation involves less bone removal and hence may prevent damage to adjacent vital structures. The cyst cavity is then open for inspection as it heals, but the cavity may be difficult for the patient to clean. It also has the disadvantage that only a portion of the cyst lining is available for histological analysis.

5.26 CDE

Monocryl, Vicryl and Vicryl Rapide are all types of resorbable suture.

5.27 **An incisional biopsy is indicated in the diagnosis of which of the following lesions?**

   A   Squamous cell carcinoma on the lateral border of the tongue

   B   Fibroepithelial polyp on the buccal mucosa

   C   Capillary haemangioma on the lower lip

   D   Sublingual keratosis

   E   A palpable lump in the submandibular gland

5.28 **Identify the sutures labelled i–iii in the figure. Choose from the list of options below.**

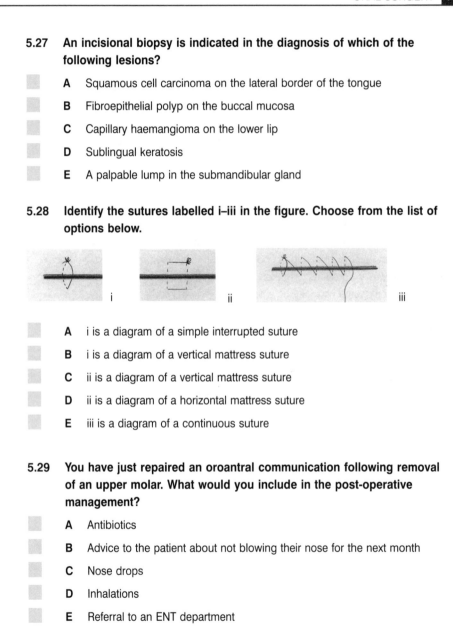

       i   ii   iii

   A   i is a diagram of a simple interrupted suture

   B   i is a diagram of a vertical mattress suture

   C   ii is a diagram of a vertical mattress suture

   D   ii is a diagram of a horizontal mattress suture

   E   iii is a diagram of a continuous suture

5.29 **You have just repaired an oroantral communication following removal of an upper molar. What would you include in the post-operative management?**

   A   Antibiotics

   B   Advice to the patient about not blowing their nose for the next month

   C   Nose drops

   D   Inhalations

   E   Referral to an ENT department

5.27 AD

Incisional biopsies are indicated for oral squamous cell carcinomas and sublingual keratosis. A fibroepithelial polyp on the buccal mucosa should be removed in its entirety – hence an excisional biopsy is indicated. A capillary haemangioma should not have a biopsy carried out on it. A lump in the submandibular gland may be investigated by fine needle aspiration but not an open incisional biopsy.

5.28 ABC

i is a simple interrupted suture, commonly used for intra and extra oral wounds. ii is a horizontal mattress suture often used in bleeding tooth sockets. iii is a continuous suture, which has the advantage of being quicker to do than multiple interrupted sutures. However, care must be taken when tying the knots of a continuous suture because if they come undone, the whole suture line will come undone.

5.29 ACD

After the closure of an oro-antral communication a patient should be advised to avoid blowing their nose until the surgical site has healed, usually 10–14 days. Antibiotics, nose drops and inhalations are often prescribed. The repair usually heals without on-going sinus problems, so patients do not usually need to be referred to ENT.

5.30 **Which of the following could occur following a fracture of the zygoma?**

   A   Anosmia

   B   Bruising in the ipsilateral upper buccal sulcus

   C   Anaesthesia of the ipsilateral cheek

   D   Epistaxis

   E   Diplopia

5.31 **Which of the following are common signs and symptoms of a fracture of the zygomatic arch?**

   A   Limitation of mouth opening

   B   Deviation of the mandible on opening to the ipsilateral side

   C   Deviation of the mandible on opening to the contralateral side

   D   Diplopia

   E   Epistaxis

5.32 **Regarding operating on the submandibular gland:**

   A   Damage to the lingual nerve will cause loss of sensation to the posterior third of the tongue

   B   The submandibular gland wraps around the posterior border of mylohyoid

   C   The buccal branch of the facial nerve is at risk of surgical trauma

   D   The hypoglossal nerve is seen to loop under the submandibular duct

   E   The safest site for an incision is on the lower border of the mandible to prevent damage to the facial nerve

5.30   BCDE

Signs and symptoms of a fractured zygoma include: anaesthesia or paraesthesia of the cheek, side of nose and upper lip due to damage to the infra-orbital nerve; epistaxis (nose bleed) as blood drains out of the maxillary antrum; and diplopia (double vision), usually due to oedema around the eye and bruising of the upper buccal sulcus. Anosmia or loss of smell does not usually occur.

5.31 AB

Fractured zygomatic arches frequently cause difficulty in mandibular movements due to the fractured pieces impinging on the temporalis muscle and underlying mandibular coronoid process. When patients try to open their mouth their lower jaw will deviate towards the fractured side as the mandible will not translate in the normal manner. Epistaxis or diplopia does not usually occur unless there are other associated injuries.

5.32 B

The lingual nerve supplies the anterior two-thirds of the tongue and the glossopharyngeal nerve supplies the posterior third of the tongue. Incisions are usually sited two finger widths below the lower border of the mandible to avoid damage to the marginal mandibular branch of the facial nerve, the branch at greatest risk of damage during surgery of this gland. The lingual nerve loops around the submandibular duct, not the hypoglossal nerve.

5.33   **Regarding the muscles of mastication:**

A   The temporalis can be divided into anterior, middle and posterior fibres, all of which carry out the same movements

B   The anterior and middle fibres contribute to elevation of the mandible

C   The middle and posterior fibres contribute to elevation of the mandible

D   The anterior and middle fibres contribute to retrusion of the mandible

E   The posterior fibres contribute to retrusion of the mandible

5.34   **Regarding the ligaments of the temporomandibular joint:**

A   The temporomandibular ligament is related to the lateral aspect of the joint

B   The stylomandibular ligament is a remnant of the deep cervical fascia as it passes lateral to the parotid gland

C   The stylohyoid ligament extends from the tip of the styloid process to the lingula

D   The sphenomandibular ligament extends from the spine of the sphenoid to the lingula

E   The sphenomandibular ligament is a remnant of Meckel's cartilage

5.35   **Regarding the temporomandibular joint:**

A   The articular surfaces of the joint are covered with fibrocartilage

B   The articular surfaces are covered with hyaline cartilage

C   The articular disc is composed of hyaline cartilage

D   The middle part of the disc is the vascular area

E   The disc attaches to the articular capsule anteriorly

5.33 BE

The temporalis muscle can be divided into three parts which carry out different movements. The posterior fibres retract the mandible, and the remaining fibres of the muscle elevate the mandible.

5.34 ADE

The stylomandibular ligament is a remnant of the deep cervical fascia as it passes medial to the parotid gland. The stylohyoid ligament extends from the tip of the styloid process to the angle of the mandible.

5.35 A

The articular surfaces of the temporomandibular joint are covered with fibrocartilage, and the articular disc is also made of fibrocartilage. The middle part of the disc is avascular. The disc attaches to the anterior margin of the articular eminence, the articular margin of the condyle and the lateral pterygoid muscle.

6

Child Dental Health
and Orthodontics

6.1   Regarding dento-alveolar trauma:

A   Concussion means injury to the supporting tissues of a tooth with displacement

B   Concussion means injury to the supporting tissues of a tooth without displacement

C   Luxation means displacement of a tooth

D   Subluxation means loosening of a tooth in its socket without displacement

E   Subluxation means loosening of a tooth in its socket with a dento-alveolar fracture

6.2   Which of the following could cause a crossbite?

A   Thumb-sucking habit

B   Skeletal discrepancy

C   Cleft lip and palate

D   Amelogenesis imperfecta

E   Osteogenesis imperfecta

6.3   Which of the following factors would increase a child's risk for caries?

A   Coming from an affluent family

B   Having a poorly educated mother

C   High caries rate in siblings

D   Exposure to fluoride

E   Having a decreased salivary flow rate

6.1 BCD

Luxation means displacement of a tooth. It is used to describe displacement in any direction except apically and occlusally, in which case the displacement is known as intrusion and extrusion, respectively. Concussion means that the tooth is traumatised, but it has not moved in its socket. Subluxation is used to describe loosening of a tooth without displacement, despite the fact that the word subluxation actually means partial displacement.

6.2 ABC

Anything that may alter the normal relationship of maxillary to mandibular teeth may cause a crossbite, eg a skeletal discrepancy or a cleft palate. Prolonged thumb sucking may cause tilting of the teeth and narrowing of the maxillary arch, which can also result in a crossbite.

6.3 BCE

To determine the risk status of a child for caries, socio-demographic, dental and other factors must all be considered. Children with a high risk for caries are usually in the lower socio-economic groups with poorly educated parents. The caries experience of siblings should also be taken into consideration, as a high caries experience would put the child at greater risk. Exposure to fluoride decreases the risk of caries whereas a decreased salivary flow rate increases the caries risk.

6.4 **Which of the following situations would be appropriate for using fissure sealants?**

A On the deciduous molars of a child with extensive caries in their deciduous teeth

B On the permanent molars of a child with extensive caries in their deciduous teeth

C In a caries-free child

D In a child with an impairment

E Only within 24 months of the eruption of the tooth in question

6.5 **Which of the following methods of topical fluoride application are appropriate in an 8-year-old child (who lives in an area with < 0.3 ppm of fluoride in the water supply)?**

A Toothpaste with 500 ppm of fluoride

B Toothpaste with 1000 ppm of fluoride

C 0.05% fluoride mouthwash daily

D 0.05% fluoride mouthwash weekly

E 0.5 mg fluoride tablets daily

6.6 **The force required to bodily move a single-rooted tooth is about:**

A 5–10 g

B 10–50 g

C 50–100 g

D 100–150 g

E 150–500 g

6.4   BD

Fissure sealants are not normally used on deciduous teeth. They are used on permanent teeth and do not need to be placed within a limited time of the tooth erupting. They should be considered for children who have extensive caries in their primary dentition, children with impairments and in children whose general health would be jeopardised by either the development of oral disease or the need for dental treatment.

6.5   BC

Mouthwashes are contra-indicated in young children, but a child of 8 years should be able to use them. The ideal is 0.05% fluoride daily, but it may be substituted by a 0.2% mouthwash once a week. A fluoride concentration of 500 ppm in toothpaste for an 8-year-old is too low, it should 1000 ppm. Fluoride 1 mg tablets are appropriate for 8-year-olds.

6.6   D

The force required to move a tooth bodily is greater than that required to tip a tooth as it is distributed over a greater area of the periodontal ligament. For a single-rooted tooth about 100–150 g force is required for bodily movement. Larger forces are required for multi-rooted teeth.

6.7   Excessive force during orthodontic treatment may result in:

A   Root resorption

B   Mobility of teeth

C   Increase in anchorage

D   Increased caries rate

E   Delayed tooth movement

6.8   Advantages of removable appliance therapy include:

A   They are easier to clean than fixed appliances

B   Intermaxillary traction is possible

C   Groups of teeth can be moved together

D   Speech is rarely affected

E   Bodily tooth movements are possible

6.9   Which of the following statements are true?

A   Balancing extractions are removal of the same tooth (or adjacent tooth) on the same side in the opposing arch

B   Balancing extractions are removal of the same tooth (or adjacent tooth) in the same arch on the other side

C   Compensating extractions are removal of the same tooth (or adjacent tooth) on the same side in the opposing arch

D   Compensating extractions are removal of the same tooth (or adjacent tooth) in the same arch on the other side

6.7 ABE

One of the complications of orthodontic treatment is root resorption, both lateral and apical. This occurs more frequently when greater forces are used. Teeth may also become mobile and tooth movement can be delayed rather than speeded up. Use of excessive force does not cause an increase in caries rate but may result in a decrease in anchorage.

6.8 AC

Intermaxillary traction is not possible with removable appliances. Removable appliances tip teeth rather than move them bodily. They often affect speech more than a fixed appliance as the baseplate is bulky and encroaches on the tongue space.

6.9 BC

Balancing extractions refers to extractions on the other side of the arch and compensating extractions to extractions in the opposing arch.

6.10 **Which of the following are normal cephalometric values for Caucasians?**

A   SNA: 79° ± 3°

B   Upper central incisor to maxillary plane:109° ± 6°

C   ANB: 3° ± 2°

D   MMPA: 35° ± 4°

E   MMPA: 27° ± 4°

6.11 **Which of the following landmarks are used to describe the various cephalometric planes?**

A   S to N: Frankfort plane

B   Po to Or: Frankfort plane

C   Po to Or: Mandibular plane

D   PNS to ANS: Maxillary plane

E   PNS to ANS: Mandibular plane

6.12 **Which descriptions of the following commonly used cephalometric landmarks are correct?**

A   Sella is the anterior wall of sella turcica

B   Nasion is the most anterior point on the fronto-nasal suture

C   Orbitale is the most superior point on the orbital rim

D   Porion is the most anterior point on the mandibular symphysis

E   Menton is the most inferior point on the mandibular symphysis

6.10 BCE

Normal values are as follows:

- SNA: 81° ± 3°
- SNB: 79° ± 3°
- MMPA: 27° ± 4°

6.11 BD

Go to Me: Mandibular plane.

6.12 BE

Sella is the central point of the sella turcica, and orbitale is the most inferior point on the orbital rim. The pogonion is the most anterior point on the mandibular symphysis, whereas porion is the uppermost anterior point on the external auditory meatus.

6.13 A 14-year-old boy arrives at your surgery with an absent upper right permanent canine. The upper left permanent canine erupted 12 months ago. Which of the following observations would suggest that the upper right canine was buccally impacted?

A A palpable bulge in the anterior palate on the right

B A proclined permanent upper right lateral incisor

C A buccally situated upper canine on the other side

D A retroclined permanent upper right lateral incisor

E A buccal bulge in the alveolus in the region of the canine on the right hand side

6.14 A 13-year-old girl attends your dental practice. She is a thumb sucker. What type of malocclusion would she be likely to have?

A Anterior openbite

B Posterior openbite

C Posterior crossbite

D Increased overbite

E Decreased overbite

6.15 A 15-year-old girl attends your surgery with a midline diastema. Which of the following could possibly be a cause of a midline diastema?

A Normal development

B Midline conical supernumerary

C Hypodontia

D Prominent lingual fraenum

E Microdontia

6.13 BE

The majority of impacted canines are palatal and unilateral. A proclined lateral incisor may indicate the unerupted canine is buccal, as the unerupted tooth pushes the root tip of the lateral incisor palatally and its crown buccally. A palpable bulge buccally may also indicate that the tooth is lying buccally. A buccally impacted or erupted canine on one side has no bearing on the other as impactions are not symmetrical.

6.14 ACE

Thumb sucking usually leads to proclination of the upper incisors and retroclination of the lower incisors which can cause a decreased overbite or an anterior open bite. A posterior crossbite often occurs due to over-activity of the buccinator muscles.

6.15 BCE

Diastemas due to normal development (physiological spacing) are likely to close spontaneously with eruption of the permanent canine (11–13 years). A prominent lingual fraenum will have no bearing on the position of the upper incisors.

6.16 **Regarding pulp treatment of primary teeth:**

A   Pulpotomy means the removal of the entire coronal and radicular pulp

B   Beechwood creosote is used for one-visit pulpotomies on vital pulps

C   Formocresol is used for vital pulpotomies

D   15.5% ferric sulphate can be used instead of beechwood creosote

E   Cvek's pulpotomy is done for vital pulps

6.17 **Which of the following factors make restoring deciduous teeth different from restoring permanent teeth?**

A   Crowns of deciduous teeth are more bulbous than permanent teeth

B   Crowns of permanent teeth are more bulbous than deciduous teeth

C   The enamel is laid down in a more orderly fashion in deciduous teeth

D   Deciduous teeth have broader contact points than permanent teeth

E   Deciduous teeth have narrower contact points than permanent teeth

6.18 **Which of the following types of behaviour management techniques are used when treating children in the dental surgery?**

A   Tell, show, do

B   Modelling

C   Sensitisation

D   Positive reinforcement

E   Behaviour shaping

6.16   C

Pulpectomy means the removal of the entire coronal and radicular pulp. Beechwood creosote is used for devitalising pulpotomies. Formoscresol is used for vital pulpotomies, and 15.5% ferric sulphate can be used instead. Cvek's pulpotomy is carried out on permanent teeth, usually incisors, in an effort to allow apex formation to occur following trauma to the pulp.

6.17   AD

The crowns of deciduous teeth are more bulbous than permanent teeth and their contact points are wider. The enamel on deciduous teeth is thinner. The enamel is laid down in a more orderly fashion in permanent teeth, hence they do not need to be etched for as long as deciduous teeth.

6.18   ABDE

Desensitisation, not sensitisation, is a behaviour management method used for children with pre-existing fears.

6.19   Regarding eruption dates:

   A   Deciduous maxillary upper central incisors erupt at about 7 months

   B   Deciduous mandibular canines erupt at about 12–16 months

   C   Deciduous mandibular second molars erupt at about 21–30 months

   D   Deciduous maxillary second molars erupt at about 30–34 months

   E   Permanent maxillary first premolars erupt at about 10–11 years

6.20   Which of the following statements are correct?

   A   The crowns of the permanent maxillary central incisors start to calcify at 3–4 months in utero

   B   The permanent maxillary central incisors erupt at about age 7–8 years and the root formation is complete at about age 10

   C   The crowns of the permanent maxillary canines start to calcify at birth

   D   The permanent mandibular second molars erupt at about age 12–13 and root formation is complete at about age 14–15

   E   The crowns of the maxillary first premolars start to form at about 18–24 months

6.21   Which of the following may be signs that a patient is not wearing their removable orthodontic appliance?

   A   Difficulty inserting the appliance

   B   Poor speech

   C   Springs very loose at next visit

   D   No evidence of wear on the appliance

   E   Poor fit

6.19 ACE

Deciduous mandibular canines erupt at about 16–20 months. Deciduous mandibular and maxillary second molars erupt at about 21–30 months.

6.20 BDE

The crowns of the permanent maxillary central incisors start to calcify at 3–4 months after birth. The crowns of the permanent maxillary canines start to calcify at about age 4–5 months.

6.21 ABDE

All are signs that a patient is not wearing their appliance except that springs are usually active if the appliance has not been used.

6.22   A mother telephones your dental practice. Her 10-year-old daughter
        has a knocked-out upper central incisor following a roller skating
        accident. The mother is not sure how to re-implant the tooth, so you
        advise her to attend the practice with the daughter and tooth. Which
        of the following storage media are suitable for the avulsed tooth?

        A   Milk

        B   Chlorhexidine mouthwash

        C   Placing the tooth in the buccal sulcus of the daughter's mouth

        D   Saline or contact lens solution

        E   Cold water

6.23   The following are often seen in children with non-accidental injuries:

        A   Bruises of differing ages present at the same time

        B   Injuries that appear consistent with the explanation of how they occurred

        C   Fraenal tears

        D   Injuries in the head and neck region

        E   Older children are often involved

6.22 ACD

Ideally the tooth should be re-implanted as soon as possible, but if no-one on site is capable of doing it then they should bring the tooth to the surgery for re-implantation. The ideal storage medium should be as physiological as possible. Hence the tooth should not be placed in chlorhexidine mouthwash. Cold water is not ideal as it is hypotonic and may result in lysis of the periodontal ligament cells.

6.23 ACD

Non-accidental injuries occur in the head and neck region in 50% of cases. Patients often have bruises of differing ages and often present late for treatment. Injuries often appear inconsistent with the explanation of how they occurred. Injuries are often inflicted on younger rather than older children.

7

Therapeutics

7.1 **Which of the following statements are correct?**

A Flumazenil is a benzodiazepine agonist

B Flumazenil is a benzodiazepine antagonist

C Benzodiazepines are commonly used anxiolytic drugs

D Benzodiazepines may be used in the treatment of epilepsy

E Carbamazepine is a benzodiazepine

7.2 **Which of the following statements are correct?**

A Lidocaine 0.2% with 1:80 000 adrenaline (epinephrine) is a commonly used dental local anaesthetic

B Lidocaine has a longer lasting anaesthetic effect than bupivacaine

C Plain lidocaine provides more pronounced dental anaesthesia than lidocaine with adrenaline

D Prilocaine 3% with 0.03 IU/ml felypressin is a commonly used dental local anaesthetic

E Lidocaine must be stored at 4 °C

7.3 **Which of the following statements are correct?**

A A 2.2 ml cartridge of 2% lidocaine and 1:80 000 adrenaline contains 4.4 mg of lidocaine

B Lidocaine and prilocaine contain an ester group

C Esters are less likely to cause allergic reactions than amides

D Amide local anaesthetics are metabolised by the liver

E Prilocaine has a much higher toxicity than lidocaine

7.1 BCD

Benzodiazepines are central nervous system depressants and act as sedatives, hypnotics, anxiolytics and anti-convulsants. Flumazenil is a benzodiazepine antagonist, commonly used to reverse the action of midazolam. Although having a name that sounds similar to benzodiazepine, carbamazepine is not a benzodiazepine.

7.2 D

Lidocaine 2% with 1:80 000 adrenaline is a commonly used dental local anaesthetic. It has a more pronounced effect than lidocaine alone as adrenaline causes vasoconstriction, which prevents the solution dispersing away from the site of action. Bupivacaine is a longer lasting local anaesthetic than lidocaine.

7.3 D

A 2% solution will contain 20 mg/ml, so a 2.2 ml cartridge contains 44 mg of lidocaine. Lidocaine and prilocaine contain an amide group, and as such are less likely to cause an allergic reaction than an ester-containing local anaesthetic. Lidocaine has higher toxicity than prilocaine.

7.4 **Which of the following drugs interact with warfarin and may increase a patient's international normalised ratio (INR)?**

A   Fluconazole

B   Vitamin K

C   Metronidazole

D   Erythromycin

E   Oral contraceptives

7.5 **Non-steroidal anti-inflammatory drugs (NSAIDs) are best avoided in:**

A   Patients with a history of gastric bleeding

B   Asthmatic patients

C   Patients who are hypersensitive to aspirin

D   Children under the age of 6 years due to the possibility of Reye's syndrome

E   Patients on paracetamol

7.6 **Penicillins:**

A   Are the antibiotic of choice for anaerobic infections

B   Interfere with bacterial cell wall synthesis

C   Are bacteriocidal

D   Are antagonistic to tetracycline

E   Rarely cause allergic reactions

7.4 ACD

Fluconazole, erythromycin and metronidazole may interact with warfarin and potentiate its action. The oral contraceptive pill and vitamin K may interact with warfarin, but they reduce its effect hence lowering the INR.

7.5 ABCD

NSAIDs should be avoided in any patient with a history of hypersensitivity to aspirin or any other NSAID. They should also be avoided in patients with gastric/duodenal ulceration, and if it is necessary to prescribe them, then they should be given in conjunction with a selective inhibitor of cyclo-oxygenase–2 or gastroprotective treatment. Reye's syndrome can be caused by patients under the age of 16 years taking aspirin and hence it should be avoided in children. Patients on paracetamol can take NSAIDs as well as they have different modes of action and do not interact.

7.6 BCD

The penicillins all act by interfering with bacterial cell wall synthesis, by inhibiting cross-linking of the mucopeptides in the cell wall and as such are bacteriocidal. Bacteria are attacked when cells are dividing and so in theory antibiotics that are bacteriostatic would decrease the efficacy of bacteriocidal drugs. However, this doesn't often cause a problem but tetracycline and penicillin are antagonistic and should not be used at the same time. Metronidazole is the antibiotic of choice for anaerobic infections.

7.7 What are the appropriate drugs and dosages for use in the following emergencies?

A In suspected anaphylaxis – 1:1000 adrenaline 0.5 ml intravenously

B In suspected anaphylaxis – chlorphenamine 10 mg in 1 ml intramuscularly

C In a suspected angina attack – glyceryl trinitrate intramuscularly

D In a suspected diabetic hypoglycaemic collapse where the patient is unconscious – glucagon 10 mg intramuscularly

E In a suspected diabetic hypoglycaemic collapse where the patient is unconscious – 50 ml of 20% glucose intravenously

7.8 Paracetamol is:

A Anti-pyretic

B Anti-inflammatory

C Locally acting

D Hepatotoxic in overdose

E Taken in doses of 500 mg –1 g four times a day

7.9 Which of the following drugs and doses are commonly used in the treatment of atypical facial pain?

A Amitriptyline 10–25 mg daily

B Nortriptyline 10–25 mg daily

C Protirelin 10–25 mg daily

D Fluoxetine 20 mg daily

E Flumazenil 20 mg daily

7.7   BE

In suspected anaphylaxis 0.5 ml of 1:1000 adrenaline is given intramuscularly as is chlorphenamine 10 mg in 1 ml (also intramuscularly). In an angina attack glyceryl trinitrate is usually administered sublingually. In a hypoglycaemic collapse glucagon 1 mg is given intramuscularly and/or 50 ml of 20% glucose intravenously.

7.8   ADE

Paracetamol is a centrally acting analgesic with anti-pyretic properties. Unlike the NSAIDs it does not have anti-inflammatory properties. It is hepatotoxic in high doses.

7.9   ABD

Amitriptyline and nortriptyline are both tricyclic antidepressants and are used in the treatment of atypical facial pain. Fluoxetine is a selective serotonin reuptake inhibitor and also used in the treatment of facial pain. Protirelin is a hypothalamic-releasing hormone which stimulates the release of thyrotrophin from the pituitary gland and so is not used for treatment of atypical facial pain. Flumazenil is a benzodiazepine antagonist used to reverse the central sedative effects of benzodiazepines.

7.10   Which of the following are anti-fungal drugs?

A   Miconazole

B   Aciclovir

C   Chlorhexidine

D   Nystatin

E   Itraconazole

7.11   Which of the following must always be included in a prescription?

A   The name and address of the prescriber

B   The age of the patient

C   The date of prescription

D   The dose of the drug in numbers and words

E   The address of the patient

7.12   Which of the following drug doses and concentrations are correct for using in an anaphylactic reaction?

A   Adrenaline 0.5 ml of 1:100 intramuscularly

B   Adrenaline 0.5 ml of 1:1000 intramuscularly

C   Hydrocortisone sodium succinate 2 mg intravenously

D   Hydrocortisone sodium succinate 20 mg intravenously

E   Hydrocortisone sodium succinate 200 mg intravenously

7.10   ADE

Miconazole is an imidazole anti-fungal drug, Nystatin is a polyene anti-fungal drug and itraconazole is a triazole anti-fungal. Aciclovir is an anti-viral drug and chlorhexidine is an antiseptic.

7.11   ACE

The name and address of the prescriber, the date of prescription and the address of the patient must be included. It is desirable to include the age and date of birth of the patient, but this is a legal requirement for only prescription-only medicines for patients under 12 years of age. The drug dose only needs to be put in words and figures if it is a controlled drug.

7.12   BE

Appropriate treatment of a suspected anaphylactic attack involves 0.5–1 ml of a 1:1000 solution of adrenaline administered intramuscularly. Hydrocortisone sodium succinate 200 mg intravenously should also be given.

7.13 Which of the following drugs cause lichenoid reaction?

A β-Blockers

B Nifedipine

C Allopurinol

D Phenytoin

E Anti-malarials

7.14 Which of the following drugs cause a dry mouth?

A Heavy metal poisoning

B Atropine

C Tricyclic antidepressants

D Anti-emetics

E Anti-malarials

7.15 You have prescribed oral metronidazole. What instructions do you need to give the patient?

A Take the tablets twice a day

B Take the tablets three times a day

C Take the tablets until the pain has subsided

D Avoid drinking alcohol while taking the tablets

E Take the whole course as prescribed

7.13 ACE

β-Blockers, anti-malarials and allopurinol cause lichenoid reactions. Phenytoin and nifedipine cause gingival hyperplasia.

7.14 BCD

Anti-malarials cause lichenoid reactions. Atropine is an anti-muscarinic drug (formerly known as anti-cholinergics). It reduces gastric and salivary secretions, and hence causes a dry mouth. Some tricyclics and anti-emetics also cause dry mouth.

7.15 BDE

Oral metronidazole is usually prescribed as 200 mg or 400 mg tablets taken three times a day. It is important that patients do not drink alcohol while taking metronidazole as the two will interact. Antibiotic courses should be completed as prescribed and not stopped when pain subsides.

7.16 **Which of the following are correct regarding the action of local anaesthetic agents?**

A   Local anaesthetics block hydrogen channels

B   Local anaesthetics block sodium channels

C   Local anaesthetics block potassium channels

D   Local anaesthetics have membrane-stabilising properties

E   Local anaesthetics have membrane-activating properties

7.17 **Aspirin:**

A   Is an NSAID

B   Prevents the synthesis of prostaglandin E_3

C   Is anti-pyretic

D   May cause gastric mucosal irritation and bleeding

E   Is commonly used as an analgesic for children

7.18 **Which of the following antibiotic cover regimens are appropriate for patients with cardiac pacemakers who require dental extractions?**

A   Under local anaesthesia with 3 g amoxicillin orally, 1 hour before the procedure

B   Under local anaesthesia with 600 mg clindamycin orally, 1 hour before the procedure

C   Under local anaesthesia with 600 mg clindamycin orally, 1 hour before the procedure and 300 mg clindamycin orally 6 hours later

D   Under general anaesthesia with 1 g amoxicillin and 120 mg gentamycin intravenously at induction

E   Under general anaesthesia 1 g amoxicillin and 120 mg gentamycin intravenously at induction with 500 mg amoxicillin orally 6 hours later

7.16 BD

Local anaesthetics work by producing reversible inhibition of impulses in peripheral nerves by virtue of their membrane-stabilising properties. They act by blocking sodium channels and preventing membrane depolarisation.

7.17 ACD

Aspirin is an NSAID which acts by preventing the synthesis of prostaglandin E_2. It is anti-pyretic by virtue of its action on the hypothalamus and inhibition of prostaglandin synthesis, which is a mediator of febrile response to infections. It should not be used for children as it can cause Reye's syndrome.

7.18 All statements are false

Patients who have cardiac pacemakers do not require prophylactic antibiotic cover for dental extractions.

7.19 Patients on oral anticoagulants:

A   Carry a blue warning card

B   Must wear a MedicAlert bracelet

C   Have their anti-coagulation monitored by regular blood tests to measure their INR

D   Have a target therapeutic range of INR 2–3

E   Must stop their anticoagulants 3 days prior to tooth extractions

7.20 Which of the following drugs can be safely prescribed in pregnancy?

A   Metronidazole

B   Paracetamol

C   Prilocaine

D   Miconazole

E   Amoxycillin

7.21 Which of the following drugs commonly cause gingival hyperplasia?

A   Nifedipine

B   Phenytoin

C   Ciclosporin

D   Diltiazem

E   Carbamazepine

7.19 C

Blue warning cards are steroid cards. MedicAlert bracelets are not necessarily worn by patients on warfarin, although some may wear them depending on their medical history. Patients on anticoagulants have a target range that their INR is meant to stay between. This will vary depending on the condition for which they are taking the anticoagulants, for example the therapeutic range for prophylaxis of deep vein thrombosis is 2–2.5 and the therapeutic range for patients with prosthetic heart valves is 3.5. Depending on a patient's INR it may not be necessary to stop their anticoagulants prior to extractions, as many extractions can be carried out safely without altering the warfarin dose.

7.20 BE

Care must always be taken when prescribing drugs during pregnancy. Metronidazole, prilocaine and miconazole should be avoided as far as possible.

7.21 ABCD

Carbamazepine causes erythema multiforme, whereas the others may cause gingival hyperplasia.

7.22 Which of the following are well known side effects of the named drugs?

A Nifedipine may cause gingival hyperplasia

B Gentamicin may cause 'red man syndrome'

C Carbamazepine may cause a skin rash

D Clindamycin may cause pseudomembranous colitis

E Aspirin may cause Reye's syndrome

7.23 Which of the following are complications of long-term steroid therapy?

A Striae

B Hypotension

C Adrenal suppression

D Osteoporosis

E Weight loss

7.24 Which of the following antibiotic cover regimens are appropriate for adult patients with prosthetic heart valves who require dental extractions?

A Under local anaesthesia with 3 mg amoxicillin orally, 1 hour before the procedure

B Under local anaesthesia with 600 mg clindamycin orally, 1 hour before the procedure

C Under local anaesthesia with 600 mg clindamycin orally, 1 hour before the procedure and 300 mg clindamycin orally 6 hours later

D Under general anaesthesia with 1 g amoxicillin with 120 mg gentamicin intravenously at induction

E Under general anaesthesia with 1 mg amoxicillin and 120 mg gentamicin intravenously at induction with 500 mg amoxicillin orally 6 hours later

7.22 ACDE

Vancomycin causes 'red man syndrome'.

7.23 ACD

Long-term steroid therapy has many complications including striae on the skin, hypertension, adrenal suppression, osteoporosis and weight gain.

7.24 B

The antibiotic regimen of choice for adult patients with prosthetic heart valves requiring a dental extraction depends on whether the procedure is to be done under local or general anaesthesia. For local anaesthesia, 3 g oral amoxicillin is used, or if the patient is allergic to penicillin 600 mg clindamycin is given. No further dosing is required.

For treatment under general anaesthesia the regimens all involve intravenous drugs administration. Amoxicillin 1 g and gentamicin 120 mg is given at induction followed by 500 mg amoxicillin 6 hours later. If the patient is allergic to penicillin, vancomycin 1 g by slow intravenous infusion and 120 mg gentamicin at induction, or teicoplanin 400 mg and gentamycin 120 mg at induction, or clindamycin 600 mg at induction is given.

7.25 Which of the following may be signs and symptoms of lidocaine overdose:

  A Light headedness

  B Tachycardia

  C Convulsions

  D Hypertension

  E Hyperventilation

7.26 Erythromycin:

  A Is a macrolide drug

  B Is active against some penicillinase resistant staphylococci

  C Is active against *Chlamydia* and mycoplasmas

  D Should not be used during pregnancy

  E Is given to an adult in a regimen of 250–500 mg three times daily for 5 days

7.27 Tetracyclines:

  A Are broad-spectrum antibiotics

  B Are absorbed better when taken with milk

  C May be used as a mouthwash in a dose of 25 mg dissolved in a little water and held in the mouth

  D Cause intrinsic staining of teeth

  E Cause extrinsic staining of teeth

7.25 AC

Signs and symptoms of lidocaine overdose include light headedness, confusion, twitching leading to convulsions, hypotension, bradycardia and depression of respiration.

7.26 ABC

Erythromycin is a macrolide-type drug. It is safe to use in pregnancy and is prescribed in a regimen of 250–500 mg four times daily for 5 days. It is active against some penicillinase resistant staphylococci, although many are now becoming resistant to it.

7.27 AD

Tetracyclines are broad-spectrum antibiotics which bind to calcium and hence get deposited in teeth and bones. They cause intrinsic staining of teeth if taken during tooth development, and as such should not be prescribed to pregnant women and to children up to 12 years of age. Their absorption is decreased when taken with milk. Tetracycline mouthwash is used to reduce secondary infection when patients have oral ulceration. A 250 mg capsule is broken and dissolved in a little water and used as a mouthwash three times daily.

8

Dental
Materials

8.1 Which of the following statements are correct?

A Thermal diffusivity is the ability of a material to conduct heat

B Wear is abrasion (with or without a chemical) of a substance

C Resilience is a measure of how hard it is to bend a material

D Creep is the slow dimensional change under load

E Stress is the internal force per unit cross-sectional area acting on a material

8.2 Regarding dental amalgam:

A It is a mixture of silver alloy and mercury

B It can be composed of spherical particles, irregular particles or a mixture of the two

C Gamma–2 is the name given to the silver–mercury product formed during amalgamation

D Dimensional change is said to be negative if an amalgam expands during setting

E Titration is the process of mixing the silver alloy and mercury

8.3 The advantages of using a high-copper amalgam over a low-copper amalgam are:

A High copper amalgam has more gamma–2 phase and is therefore stronger than low copper amalgam

B High copper amalgam has less gamma–2 phase and is therefore stronger than low copper amalgam

C High copper amalgams show less corrosion than low copper amalgams

D High copper levels prevent amalgams from expanding when contaminated with saliva

8.1 BDE

Thermal diffusivity is the rate at which temperature changes spread through materials, thermal conductivity is the ability of a material to conduct heat. Resilience is the energy absorbed by a material undergoing elastic deformation (up to its elastic limit) whereas stiffness is a measure of how hard it is to bend a material.

8.2 AB

Dental amalgam is a mixture of silver alloy and mercury. Gamma–1 is the name given to silver–mercury alloy, gamma is the name given to the silver alloy and the tin–mercury product is called gamma-2. Dimensional change is said to be negative if an amalgam contracts during setting. The process of mixing amalgam is called trituration.

8.3 BC

High-copper amalgam has almost no gamma–2 phase and is therefore stronger than low-copper amalgam, and shows less corrosion. It is the zinc in amalgam that was previously responsible for their high expansion rate when contaminated with saliva. Zinc has now been virtually eliminated from modern dental amalgams.

8.4 Regarding glass ionomers:

A The powder is an aluminosilicate glass

B They are mixed by adding the powder to the liquid incrementally

C They release fluoride

D Following initial placement they should be protected from dehydration

E They have no effect on the pulp

8.5 Regarding compomers:

A They release substantially more fluoride than glass ionomers

B Their wear resistance is less than resin composites

C They are more soluble than glass ionomers

D They are stronger than glass ionomers

E They bond to both enamel and dentine

8.6 With regard to cermets:

A They are metal reinforced glass ionomer cermets

B They are radiopaque

C They show less wear resistance than conventional glass ionomers

D They release more fluoride than conventional glass ionomers

E They are used in areas where aesthetics is not a primary consideration

8.4   ACD

Glass ionomers are based on polyacrylic acid and should be mixed by adding all the powder to the liquid in one go. They do release fluoride. Following initial setting they are sensitive to dehydration and must be protected otherwise crazing or surface cracks will appear. They cause a slight inflammatory reaction in the pulp which usually resolves in a few weeks.

8.5   BD

Compomers release about a tenth of the fluoride released by glass ionomers and are less soluble than glass ionomers. They do not bond to enamel and dentine, so an intermediate bonding system is needed.

8.6   ABE

Cermets as the name suggests are ceramic metal glass, they contain either silver or gold as the metal. They are radiopaque and show better wear resistance than glass ionomers, but release less fluoride. They are aesthetically poor and hence used when aesthetics is not the primary consideration.

8.7   Regarding zinc phosphate cements:

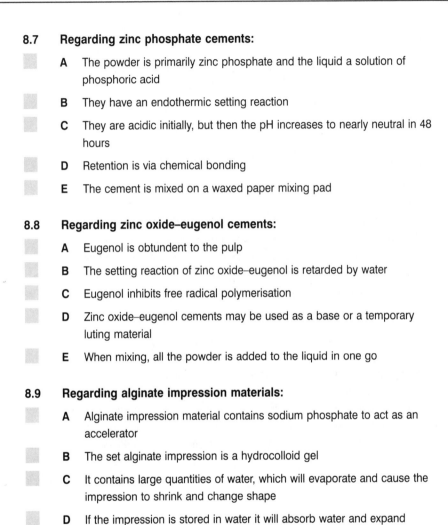

A   The powder is primarily zinc phosphate and the liquid a solution of phosphoric acid

B   They have an endothermic setting reaction

C   They are acidic initially, but then the pH increases to nearly neutral in 48 hours

D   Retention is via chemical bonding

E   The cement is mixed on a waxed paper mixing pad

8.8   Regarding zinc oxide–eugenol cements:

A   Eugenol is obtundent to the pulp

B   The setting reaction of zinc oxide–eugenol is retarded by water

C   Eugenol inhibits free radical polymerisation

D   Zinc oxide–eugenol cements may be used as a base or a temporary luting material

E   When mixing, all the powder is added to the liquid in one go

8.9   Regarding alginate impression materials:

A   Alginate impression material contains sodium phosphate to act as an accelerator

B   The set alginate impression is a hydrocolloid gel

C   It contains large quantities of water, which will evaporate and cause the impression to shrink and change shape

D   If the impression is stored in water it will absorb water and expand

E   The strength and flexibility of an alginate impression is increased if a thinner mixture (ie more water to powder) is used.

8.7 AC

Zinc phosphate cements have an exothermic setting reaction, which is why they are mixed on a cooled glass slab and not a waxed paper mixing pad. Their retention is via mechanical interlocking rather than chemical bonding.

8.8 ACD

Eugenol is a phenol derivative that can reduce pulpal irritation and has some anti-bacterial properties. Zinc oxide–eugenol cements can be used as either a base or a temporary luting cement depending on the thickness of the material. The setting reaction of zinc oxide–eugenol is accelerated by water and hence the material sets faster in the mouth than outside the mouth. Eugenol does inhibit free radical polymerisation and so may delay the setting of dental composites. When mixing the material the powder is added incrementally to the liquid.

8.9 BCD

Alginate impression materials contain sodium phosphate as a retarder. The sodium phosphate reacts with soluble calcium ions, and after all the sodium phosphate has reacted, the sodium alginate reacts with the calcium ions and calcium alginate is formed (which is a gel). The thicker the mixture of alginate (that is the greater the amount of powder to water) the less flexible and stronger the impression material will be.

8.10   Regarding impression materials:

A   Polysulphide elastomeric impression materials have higher tear resistance than alginate

B   Condensation cured silicones impression materials have shorter setting times than polysulphide elastomeric impression materials

C   Polyether impression materials absorb water under conditions of humidity as they are hydrophilic

D   The tear resistance of polysulphide impression materials is worse than the tear resistance of silicone impression materials

E   Addition-cured silicone materials shrink more than condensation-cured silicone impression materials

8.11   Cavity linings/bases are used to:

A   Protect the pulp from chemical changes

B   Protect the pulp from thermal changes

C   Provide adhesion between the tooth and restoration

D   Treat the pulp

E   Provide insulation under a metallic restoration to maximise galvanic effects

8.12   Flow of luting material is increased by:

A   Venting the restoration

B   Applying greater force when seating the restoration

C   Increasing the taper of the preparation

D   Decreasing the powder content of the cement

E   None of the above

8.10 ABC

Polyether impression materials have good dimensional stability under conditions of low humidity, but they are hydrophilic and will absorb water in humid conditions. Polysulphide impression materials have better tear resistance than silicone impression materials. As there is little or no by-product in the cross-linking reaction of addition-cured silicones they create a dimensionally stable impression compared with condensation cured materials.

8.11 ABD

Cavity linings/bases act as a protective barrier between the dentine and the restoration. They may provide thermal insulation and chemical protection. They do provide insulation under metallic restorations – to minimise galvanic action. They do not provide adhesion between the tooth and the restoration.

8.12 ACD

Decreasing the powder content of a cement will make it less viscous and so it will increase the flow of the material. Application of greater force while seating will not increase the flow of luting material. Increasing the taper allows easier escape of luting material and hence increased flow.

8.13   With respect to acid etching:

    A   It creates a microscopically rough enamel surface

    B   Following etching the etchant should be washed away with saline

    C   Enamel of deciduous teeth should be etched for a shorter time than permanent teeth

    D   The etchant is usually 20% phosphoric acid

    E   The etchant is usually applied for 15–30 seconds

8.14   Dentine bonding agents function by:

    A   Micromechanical bonds

    B   Macromechanical bonds

    C   Primary atomic bonds

    D   Secondary atomic bonds

    E   All of the above

8.15   With regard to dental composite filling materials:

    A   They consist of three phases: resin, organic filler particles and a coupling agent coated on the filler particles

    B   The resin may be based on bis-GMA (dimethacrylate) oligomers

    C   Macrofilled composites contain particles of about 0.5–2 μm in diameter

    D   They usually contain fluoride

    E   Microfilled composites are harder to polish than macrofilled composites

8.13 AE

The etchant is usually 30–50% phosphoric acid, which is applied for 15–30 seconds and creates a microscopically rough surface. As the enamel on deciduous teeth is not as regularly arranged as that on permanent teeth, they may need a longer etching time. The etchant is washed away with water not saline.

8.14 AD

Micromechanical bonds refer to the resin tags locking into the dentinal tubules. Secondary atomic bonding occurs as collagen and primers have polar groups attached to the main chains.

8.15 B

Composites consist of three phases: resin, inorganic filler particles and a coupling agent coated on the filler particles. Macrofilled composites have filler particles of around 2.5 –5 μm whereas microfilled composites have filler particles of about 0.04 μm in size. Glass ionomers, not composites, contain fluoride. The size of the filler particles determines the surface smoothness and hence microfilled composites tend to retain their shine longer and are easier to polish.

8.16 Regarding acrylic denture base materials:

A   They come in the form of a powder of polymethylmethacrylate and a liquid of ethylmethacrylate

B   An inhibitor such as benzyl peroxide is used to increase the shelf-life of the liquid

C   The material shrinks on setting

D   Heat curing leads to greater porosity in the material than cold curing

E   Ideally a high degree of conversion from monomer to polymer is desirable to increase mechanical properties of the material

8.17 Regarding the properties of casting gold alloys:

A   The gold content decreases on going from a soft type I alloy to an extra hard type IV alloy

B   The corrosion resistance increases on going from a soft type I alloy to an extra hard type IV alloy

C   The strength increases on going from a soft type I alloy to an extra hard type IV alloy

D   The ductility increases on going from a soft type I alloy to an extra hard type IV alloy

E   None of the above statements is correct

8.18 Regarding metals:

A   A molten metal should be cooled slowly to get a fine grain structure

B   Cold working will increase hardness and strength of a metal

C   Cold working will increase the brittleness of a metal

D   Internal stresses of a cold-worked metal may be removed by heat treatment at a temperature above the crystallisation temperature

E   Internal stresses of a cold-worked metal may be removed by heat treatment at a temperature below the crystallisation temperature

8.16   CE

Acrylic denture materials are usually formed of polymethylmethacrylate, which is formed by polymerisation of methylmethacrylate. They come in the form of a powder of polymethylmethacrylate and a liquid of methylmethacrylate. An inhibitor such as hydroquinone is used to increase the shelf-life of the liquid. Benzyl peroxide is the initiator, not the inhibitor. The material shrinks by about 20% on setting. Heat curing leads to less porosity in the material than cold curing. Low molecular polymer and residual monomer in the material lead to poor mechanical properties and sometime adverse tissue reactions.

8.17   AC

Type I soft casting gold alloys have about 85% gold whereas extra-hard type IV alloys have about 65% gold. This alters the properties of the alloy and the corrosion resistance and the ductility decrease on going from a soft type I alloy to an extra-hard type IV alloy.

8.18 BCE

A molten metal should be cooled rapidly to get a fine grain structure. Internal stresses of a cold-worked metal may be removed by heat treatment at a temperature well below the crystallisation temperature.

8.19   Regarding casting faults:

A   Incomplete casting could occur if the alloy is not properly melted

B   Incomplete casting may occur if there is insufficient thrust during casting

C   In order to limit porosity of a cast all casting moulds should be handled with the sprue downwards

D   Finning occurs when the investment is heated up too slowly

E   Porosity may be reduced by avoiding overheating of the alloy

8.19 ABCE

To limit porosity of a cast all casting moulds should be handled with the sprue downwards, otherwise broken bits of investment or dirt may fall down the sprue and become embedded in the casting. Handling moulds with the sprue directed downwards will limit this. Finning occurs when the investment is heated up too fast and cracks occur in the investment. Molten alloy flows into the cracks and creates fins on the casting.

9

Radiology and Radiography

9.1 **Which of the following are principles of the International Commission for Radiation Protection (ICRP)?**

A   Personal monitoring

B   Limitation

C   Screening

D   Justification

E   Optimisation

9.2 **Which of the following procedures may be undertaken by a registered dental nurse who has been appropriately trained?**

A   Reception and clerical duties

B   Taking of long cone periapical radiographs

C   Placement of temporary restorations in adults

D   Placement of temporary restorations in children

E   Impression taking

9.3 **You have taken a radiograph to assess a lower third molar for surgical removal. Which of the following radiological features would suggest that the patient would be at high risk of suffering from damage to their inferior dental nerve during the removal of the lower third molar tooth?**

A   Loss of tramlines of the inferior dental canal

B   Deviation of tramlines of the inferior dental canal

C   Widening of tramlines of the inferior dental canal

D   Narrowing of tramlines of the inferior dental canal

E   Radiopaque band across root

9.1 BDE

The ICRP recommendations are based on the principles of justification, optimisation and limitation.

- Justification – no practice should be adopted unless it produces a net benefit.
- Optimisation – all exposures should be kept as low as reasonably possible (ALARP).
- Limitation – the dose equivalent should not exceed the recommended limits.

9.2 AB

To take radiographs dental nurses should possess a certificate in dental radiography from a course conforming to the syllabus prescribed by the College of Radiographers.

9.3 ABD

Loss, narrowing and deviation of the tramlines of the inferior dental canal are all taken as evidence of association of the inferior dental nerve with a lower molar tooth. A radiolucent band across the root is also thought to indicate association of the nerve and tooth. Hence patients with these radiological features are at high risk of inferior dental nerve damage during surgical removal of lower third molar teeth.

9.4 Everyday risks to patients having radiographs taken during the course of their dental treatment include:

A Genetic stochastic effects

B Somatic stochastic effects

C Somatic deterministic effects

D Genetic deterministic effects

E None of the above

9.5 In order to limit the dose for a periapical radiograph:

A Use a lead apron

B Use a bisecting angle technique

C Use a low-speed film

D Use the optimal voltage (70 kV)

E Use a rectangular collimator

9.6 With respect to processing radiographs:

A The developer is an acidic solution

B The developer is oxidised by air and so must be changed daily

C If the film is left in the developer for too long it will result in a radiograph being too pale/light

D The lower the temperature of the developer solution the faster the film will be developed

E Fixation involves the unsensitised silver halide crystals being removed to reveal the white areas on the film

9.4   ABC

Stochastic effects are random, and can be divided into somatic and genetic. Deterministic effects are only somatic.

9.5   DE

Use of lead aprons is no longer recommended. To minimise the risk the optimal voltage (70 kV) and a fast-speed film should be used. A rectangular collimator will reduce the radiation by about 50% compared with a round collimator.

9.6   E

The developer is an alkali solution, which is oxidised by air, but is usually changed about once every 10–14 days. If the film is left in it for too long it will become too dark as more silver will be deposited on it. The higher the temperature of the developer solution the faster the process will occur – the norm is 5 minutes at 20 °C.

9.7   The stages of processing of radiographic films are:

A   Development, washing, fixation, washing, drying

B   Fixation, washing, development, washing drying

C   Washing, development, washing, fixation, drying

D   Washing, fixation, washing, development, drying

E   Washing development, fixation, washing drying

9.8   All dental practices should have a set of local rules relating to radiation protection measures. These should include:

A   The name of the radiation protection supervisor (RPS)

B   Contact details of the RPS

C   Identification and description of the controlled area

D   Arrangements for pregnant staff

E   Qualifications of the RPS

9.9   The annual dose limits under the Ionising Radiation Regulations (IRR) 1999 are:

A   General public – 2 mSv

B   Non-classified workers – 5 mSv

C   Non-classified workers – 6 mSv

D   Classified workers – 20 mSv

E   Classified workers – 60 mSv

9.7   A

When placed in the developer the sensitised silver halide crystals on the film are chemically reduced to black metallic silver. The film is then washed to remove the excess developer and placed in the fixer where the unsensitised silver halide crystals are removed, revealing the transparent parts of the image. The film is washed to remove excess fixer solution and dried.

9.8   ACD

All dental practices should have a set of local rules regarding radiation protection measures. The contact details of the RPS are not needed as they work at the practice, nor are their qualifications necessary.

9.9   CD

The annual dose limits according to IRR 1999 are:

- Classified workers – 20m Sv
- Non-classified workers – 6 mSv
- General public 1 – mSv

9.10 Film badges for monitoring and measuring radiation dosage:

A Provide a permanent record of dose received

B Should be worn outside the clothes at the level of the reproductive organs

C Can measure the type and energy of radiation encountered

D Can be assessed without processing so provide an immediate indication of exposure

E Should be replaced every 6 months

9.11 Regarding thermoluminescent dosimeters:

A They are used for monitoring radiation dose of the whole body

B They can provide a permanent record of dose received

C They use a material which absorbs radiation and then releases the energy in the form of light

D The monitor should be replaced after 1–3 months

E An advantage they have over film badges is that the monitor does not need to be replaced so frequently

9.12 The advantages of the paralleling technique of periapical radiography over the bisecting angle technique are:

A It is possible to get reproducible radiographs, even when different operators take them

B No film holder is needed

C The image produced shows little or no magnification

D The film is not coned off

E Positioning the film to take radiographs of posterior teeth is usually comfortable for the patient

9.10 ABC

Film badges are a simple and inexpensive way of recording radiation exposure. The film is usually worn outside the clothes at the level of the reproductive organs for 1–3 months. It is then processed to reveal a permanent record of the radiation dose received; no information can be gained until the film is processed, and so these badges are prone to processing errors.

9.11 ACD

Thermoluminescent dosimeters are personal monitors that contain a material that absorbs radiation and releases energy in the form of light proportional to the amount of radiation received. They are worn like a film badge and should be replaced every 1–3 months. They do not provide a permanent record, and so cannot be stored and rechecked.

9.12 ACD

As film holders are used to take periapical radiographs in the paralleling technique it is possible to get reproducible radiographs. However, positioning the film for posterior teeth may sometimes be uncomfortable.

9.13 Which of the following are indications to take a lower occlusal radiograph?

A To detect a salivary calculus in the parotid duct

B To assess fractures in the anterior body of the mandible

C To assess the buccolingual position of unerupted maxillary teeth

D To assess any buccolingual expansion of the anterior mandible by pathological lesions

E To assess the buccolingual position of unerupted mandibular third molars

9.14 Which of the following could present as multilocular radiolucent lesions in the mandible?

A Ameloblastoma

B Calcifying epithelial odontogenic tumour

C Odontogenic keratocyst

D Odontogenic myxoma

E Aneurysmal bone cyst

9.15 Which of the following lesions could present as a unilocular radiolucent lesion in the mandible?

A Dentigerous cyst

B Ameloblastoma

C Ameloblastic fibroma

D Residual cyst

E Stafne's bone cavity

9.13 BD

A lower occlusal radiograph can show a calculus in the submandibular gland duct but not in the parotid. It will show any buccolingual displacement of a symphyseal or parasymphyseal fracture of the mandible and buccolingual expansion of the mandible in the anterior mandible. It is not used to assess the buccolingual position of unerupted third molars.

9.14 ACDE

Calcifying epithelial odontogenic tumours are not usually radiolucent but are radiopaque due to the calcifying nature of the lesion.

9.15 ABCDE

Dentigerous cysts, residual cysts and Stafne's bone cavities all appear as unilocular radiolucent lesions on radiographs. Stafre's bone cavities are only seen below the inferior dental canal. Ameloblastomas although often multilocular may appear as unilocular lesions. Keratocysts are also usually multilocular, but may appear unilocular in the early stages.

9.16 **Which of the following lesions could present as a radiopaque lesion in the mandible on a dental panoramic tomogram (DPT)?**

A   Calcifying epithelial odontogenic tumour

B   Complex odontoma

C   Odontogenic fibroma

D   Cemento-osseous dysplasia

E   Submandibular gland calculus

9.17 **An ideal radiograph produces an image in which the size and shape of the object (tooth) is reproduced exactly on the film, without distortion or magnification. To produce an image as close to this which of the following principles must be applied?**

A   The distance between the tube and the film should be as small as possible

B   The distance between the film and the object should be as small as possible

C   The film should lie as near to parallel to the tooth as is possible

D   The beam should be as near to perpendicular to the tooth as possible

E   The patient should hold their breath during the taking of the radiograph

9.16 ABDE

All of the above lesions except an odontogenic fibroma could appear as radiopaque lesions in the mandible.

9.17 BCD

The distance between the tube and the film should be as large as possible. It is not necessary for patients to hold their breath during the taking of the radiograph but the patient, the tube and the film should be motionless.

10

Restorative
Dentistry

10.1 Root caries:

A   Is commoner in patients with reduced salivary flow than those with a normal salivary flow

B   Is commoner in females than in males

C   Is often managed with topical fluoride

D   Is often managed with systemic fluoride

E   May be managed by surface recontouring without a restoration

10.2 The following statements are correct:

A   The Bennett angle is the mean angle between the sagittal plane and the path of the advancing condyle during lateral excursions as viewed in the horizontal plane

B   The condylar angle is the angle between the horizontal plane and the distal slope of the articular eminence

C   The curve of Spee is the curvature of the occlusion viewed in the coronal plane

D   The curve of Wilson is the curvature of the occlusion viewed in the sagittal plane

E   Retruded contact position is the initial tooth contact when the mandible rotates around its terminal hinge axis

10.3 You are planning on restoring an upper first premolar with a porcelain restoration. Which of the following would be indications to extend the porcelain coverage over the occlusal surface of the tooth?

A   Aesthetics

B   The tooth is very short in height

C   The tooth has a large pulp cavity

D   The opposing teeth have porcelain occlusal coverage

E   The tooth is heavily restored

10.1 ACE

Root caries is a common complication of dry mouth. The lesions are often managed with topical fluoride. Systemic fluoride is not suitable as the teeth are already formed. The lesions may be managed by recontouring without placement of a restoration if they are small. Larger ones are often filled with glass ionomer cement.

10.2 ADE

The curve of Spee is the curvature of the occlusion viewed in the sagittal plane and the curve of Wilson is the curvature of the occlusion viewed in the coronal plane.

10.3 ADE

Metal occlusal coverage requires less tooth tissue removal and is therefore indicated when teeth are short and have large pulps. Porcelain occlusal coverage can be used when aesthetics is critical, when teeth are heavily restored and when they will occlude against porcelain.

10.4 **With respect to crown preparations:**

A   Resistance refers to resistance to dislodgement of the restoration under oblique forces

B   Resistance refers to resistance to dislodgement of the restoration under forces in the path of insertion of the restoration

C   Retention refers to resistance to dislodgement of the restoration under oblique forces

D   Retention refers to resistance to dislodgement of the restoration under forces in the path of insertion of the restoration

E   Height and taper of the preparation are major features in both resistance and retention

10.5 **You are restoring a vital lower first permanent molar with a deep carious cavity. In order to minimise the risk of bacteria gaining access to the pulp you could plan to:**

A   Carry out indirect pulp capping

B   Carry out direct pulp capping

C   Remove caries from the cavity wall before the cavity floor

D   Remove caries from the floor of the cavity before the cavity walls

E   Give the patient a course of antibiotics for a week

10.6 **A water spray is used with rotary instruments to:**

A   Reduce heating of the dentine

B   Reduce clogging of burs

C   Minimise movement of fluid in dentinal tubules

D   Remove debris away from operative site

E   Allow potentially infectious body fluid to be aspirated rather than creating an aerosol

10.4 ADE

Resistance refers to features that prevent removal or dislodgement of the restoration under oblique forces. Retention refers to features that that prevent removal or dislodgement of the restoration under forces along the long axis.

10.5 AC

The rationale behind indirect pulp capping is that demineralisation of the dentine precedes bacterial invasion. Hence it is possible to remove the infected dentine and treat the demineralised dentine with calcium hydroxide to encourage remineralisation.

You would not plan to do direct pulp capping as this would expose the pulp and increase the likelihood of bacteria gaining access to it. Caries should always be removed from the cavity walls first so that if an exposure is made there is a minimal load of infected material in the cavity to infect the pulp.

10.6 ABD

The water spray minimises damage to pulpal tissue via desiccation of dentine. It also helps to prevent the burs from becoming clogged. It does not minimise fluid movement in dentinal tubules. It has the detrimental effect of causing an aerosol which is potentially infectious.

10.7 **Which of the following statements about tooth surface wear are correct?**

A Attrition is tooth surface wear by non-bacterial chemical dissolution

B Abrasion is tooth surface wear by other teeth

C Abrasion is tooth surface wear by surfaces other than teeth

D Erosion is tooth surface wear by non-bacterial chemical dissolution

E Erosion is tooth surface wear by surfaces other than teeth

10.8 **Regarding non-carious tooth surface loss:**

A Abrasion is characterised by smooth wear facets

B Abrasion is the commonest type of tooth wear in young patients

C 'Cupped out' concavities are seen in patients with erosion

D Abfraction is due to stresses around the cervical margins due to flexure of teeth

E Erosion by gastric acid is usually seen on the labial aspect of the upper teeth

10.9 **Which of the following are methods of monitoring tooth surface loss?**

A Dietary sheets

B Study models

C Smith and Kidd indices

D Laser scanning

E Clinical photographs

10.7 CD

Tooth surface wear by non-bacterial chemical dissolution (dietary or gastric acid) is erosion, tooth surface wear by other teeth is attrition and tooth surface wear by surfaces other than teeth is abrasion.

10.8 CD

Attrition is the loss of tooth substance due to tooth–tooth contact and causes smooth wear facets. Abrasion is the wear of substance from an external agent, eg buccal cervical notches caused by toothbrushing, although other factors may also be operating. It is often seen in older patients. Erosion is the commonest type of tooth wear seen in young patients and when caused by gastric acid it is usually seen on the palatal aspect of the maxillary teeth.

Abfraction is due to stresses around the cervical margin due to flexure of the root and crown of the tooth. This causes minute cracks to propagate under occlusal forces.

10.9 BDE

Smith and Knight tooth indices are used to monitor tooth wear. Dietary sheets are useful to determine the cause of the problem. Laser and computer scanning of the study models and dentition – as with the other methods – taken over a period of time can be used to monitor the progression of the condition.

10.10 Which of the following may be signs and symptoms of reversible pulpitis?

A   Pain on biting

B   Sensitivity on application of heat

C   Sensitivity on application of sweet

D   Well localised pain

E   Poorly localised pain

10.11 Which of the following may be signs and symptoms of irreversible pulpitis?

A   Pain on application of heat

B   Well localised pain

C   Poorly localised pain

D   Spontaneous pain

E   Sharp, shooting pain

10.12 Which of the following statements about fluoride are true?

A   The safely tolerated dose of fluoride (ie the dose below which symptoms of toxicity are unlikely) is 1 mg/kg of body weight

B   The safely tolerated dose of fluoride is 0.5 mg/kg of body weight

C   The certainly lethal dose (ie the dose at which survival is unlikely) is 10–15 mg/kg body weight

D   The certainly lethal dose is 15–20 mg/kg body weight

E   The potentially lethal dose (ie the lowest dose associated with fatality) is 10 mg/kg body weight

10.10 BCE

Reversible pulpitis tends to cause poorly localised pain. Pain is elicited on application of hot, cold or sweet food but not on biting.

10.11 ABCD

In irreversible pulpitis there is usually spontaneous pain which may last from a few seconds to several hours. Heat causes pain which lasts long after the stimulus is withdrawn whereas cold sometimes actually relieves the pain. Irreversible pulpitis may be poorly localised if the periodontal ligament is not involved, but as soon as it is involved the patient will be able to localise the pain.

10.12 A

The potentially lethal dose of fluoride (ie the lowest dose associated with fatality) is 5 mg/kg body weight. The certainly lethal dose of fluoride (ie the dose at which survival is unlikely) is 32–64 mg/kg body weight. A person who has had a potentially lethal dose should be hospitalised.

10.13 The desirable degree of taper of a preparation to receive a cast restoration is:

A <2°

B 2–4°

C 5–7°

D 8–12°

E >12°

10.14 Regarding porcelain veneers:

A They are more durable than composite veneers in terms of colour and surface gloss

B The occlusion is not usually affected as they do not cover the palatal aspect of the teeth

C They are less likely to fracture than composite veneers

D They are more conservative of tooth tissue than crown preparations

E They usually require no preparation of the labial surface

10.15 When considering pin placement for large restorations:

A The pins should be placed in the dentinoenamel junction

B The pins should be placed in dentine

C The more pins used the stronger the restoration will be

D When more than one pin is used they must be placed parallel to each other

E Pins should be placed about 2–2.5 mm into the remaining tooth structure

10.13 C

The more parallel the walls of a restoration the greater the resistance to displacement is. However, it is not possible to achieve exactly parallel walls and so a degree of taper is acceptable, the desired taper being about 5–7°.

10.14 ABD

Porcelain is brittle and likely to fracture. Porcelain veneers usually require some preparation of tooth tissue, but they are much more conservative than crown preparations.

10.15 BE

Pins should always be placed in dentine, not at the dentinoenamel junction as the undermined enamel may fracture away. The more pins that are placed the weaker the remaining tooth and restoration will be. Pins are usually placed at an angle to the cavity walls or to other pins if possible as this increases the resistance to dislodgement.

10.16 Which of the following statements are true?

A Enamel consists of 92% hydroxyapatite crystals by weight

B Enamel is thickest where it overlies the cusps of teeth

C Diamond burs remove enamel by fracturing it

D Tungsten carbide burs remove enamel by grinding

E Stresses within a cavity preparation can be minimised by rounding the internal line angles

10.17 Which of the following are desirable properties of a matrix band for use with amalgam restorations?

A The band provides a tight fit in the cervical region

B The width of the band should be such that it extends to the marginal ridge

C The band should be see-through to allow good visibility

D The band should be thin (approx 0.05 mm)

E The band should allow contact with the adjacent tooth to be re-established

10.18 Regarding the anatomy of root canals:

A A two-rooted lower first permanent molar usually has one canal in the mesial root and one canal in the distal root

B A two-rooted lower first permanent molar usually has two canals in the distal root and one in the mesial root

C A two-rooted lower first permanent molar usually has two canals in the mesial root and one in the distal root

D The palatal root is usually the longest root in a three-rooted maxillary first permanent molar

E The mesiobuccal root is usually longer than the palatal root in a three-rooted maxillary first permanent molar

10.16 BE

Enamel consists of 96–98% hydroxyapatite crystals by weight. It is thinnest buccally and thickest over the cusps of the teeth. Diamond burs remove enamel by grinding whereas tungsten carbide burs remove enamel by fracturing it.

10.17 ADE

Matrix bands need to provide a good fit in the cervical area and should extend to 1 mm above the marginal ridge to allow for over-packing of the cavity. Matrix bands for amalgam restorations are usually metallic and do not need to be see-through. They should be smooth, thin and be adaptable so the contact point with the adjacent tooth can be re-established.

10.18 CD

Two-rooted lower first permanent molars usually have two canals in the mesial root and one in the distal root. In three-rooted maxillary first permanent molars the palatal root is usually the longest root.

10.19 **An ideal root canal filling material would have which of the following properties?**

  A   Non-irritant to the periapical tissues

  B   Be radiolucent

  C   Absorb moisture

  D   Be easily introduced into the root canal system

  E   Not visible through the dentine

10.20 **Which of the following conditions may cause a root canal treatment to fail?**

  A   Bacteria left in accessory canals

  B   Persistent infection of a root canal following treatment

  C   Presence of a coronal restoration with inadequate margins

  D   A vertical root fracture

  E   Necrotic material being left in the canal during preparation

10.21 **Obturation of a root canal system during root canal treatment aims to:**

  A   Provide a fluid-tight seal at the apical end of the root but not at the coronal end

  B   Provide a fluid-tight seal at the coronal end of the root but not at the apical end

  C   Provide a fluid-tight seal at both the apical and coronal ends of the root

  D   Seal any remaining bacteria in the root canal system

  E   Remove any remaining bacteria from the canal system

10.19 ADE

An ideal root canal filling material should be radio-opaque and should not absorb moisture – it should be impervious to moisture. The filler should not be visible through the coronal dentine.

10.20 ABCDE

All these conditions may cause failure of a root canal treatment.

10.21 CD

The aim of obturation is to provide a fluid-tight seal at both the apical and the coronal ends of the root canal. It also aims to seal any remaining bacteria in the canal system. Removal of bacteria is the aim of cleaning and preparing the canal.

10.22 Surgical endodontic treatment:

   A   Is indicated for all failed root canal treatments

   B   Is indicated when there is a broken instrument in the canal that cannot be bypassed

   C   Is indicated to prevent removal of extensive coronal restorative work

   D   Is indicated when there is evidence of a periapical radiolucency on radiographs

   E   Is contra-indicated in all multi-rooted teeth

10.23 Which of the following are features of an access cavity?

   A   It should only remove the roof of the pulp chamber over the entrance to the root canals

   B   Provide unobstructed access to the root canals

   C   Provide access in a straight line to the root canals

   D   Have parallel or convergent walls to retain a temporary restoration

   E   It is usually ovoid shaped for maxillary incisors

10.24 Which of the following are methods of obturating a canal with gutta percha?

   A   Vertical condensation

   B   Lateral trephination

   C   Thermomechanical compaction

   D   Using thermoplasticised gutta percha

   E   Vertical trephination

10.22 BC

Orthograde root canal treatment is preferable to surgical endodontics as surgery only seals over the canal that has not been re-cleaned. However, surgical endodontics may be indicated when it is not possible to bypass a broken instrument or when conventional orthograde treatment would mean removal of extensive coronal restorative work. The presence of a periapical radiolucency on radiograph is not an indication for a surgical approach. Orthograde root canal treatments can cure periapical disease. It is possible to carry out surgical endodontics on multi-rooted teeth.

10.23 BC

An access cavity should not have any of the pulp chamber roof present, as this will get in the way of the access to the root canals. The walls should also be divergent, it is not necessary to have convergent walls to retain a restoration. It is usually triangular shaped for maxillary incisors.

10.24 ACD

Trephination means to cut a circular hole and has nothing to do with obturating root canals, hence vertical and lateral trephination do not exist.

10.25 Which of the following are true of pregnancy and gingival tissue:

A Oestrogen may stimulate growth of new blood vessels and increase vascular permeability leading to hyperaemic gingivitis

B Progesterone may stimulate growth of new blood vessels and increase vascular permeability leading to hyperaemic gingivitis

C Pregnancy is associated with modified inflammatory response resulting in fibrous gingival overgrowth

D High levels of progesterone increase the immune response to plaque

E High levels of oestrogen suppresse the immune response to plaque

10.26 Which of the following bacterial species are strongly associated with adult periodontitis?

A *Porphyromonas gingivalis*

B *Bacteroides forsythus*

C *Campylobacter rectus*

D *Treponema pallidum*

E *Prevotella intermedia*

10.27 The condition "aggressive periodontitis" (AgP) is characterised by:

A Rapid attachment loss

B Underlying medical condition

C Non-familial tendency

D Rapid bone destruction

E Patients below the age of 35 years

10.25 ABE

The elevated levels of progesterone and oestrogen in pregnancy are known to modulate vascular responses and connective tissue turnover in gingival tissues, resulting in pregnancy gingivitis. The high levels of progesterone and oestrogen in pregnancy also suppress the immune response to plaque. Drugs such as phenytoin, calcium-channel blockers, immunosuppressants, eg ciclosporin, are thought to modify the inflammatory response resulting in fibrous gingival overgrowth.

10.26 ABCE

Treponema pallidum is the organism responsible for syphilis. Besides the micro-organisms listed in the question, the following are also strongly associated with adult periodontitis: *Fusobacterium nucleatum*, *Actinomycetes actinomycetemcomitans*, *Eikenella corrodens*, *Eubacterium* species and spirochaetes, eg *Treponema denticola*.

10.27 AD

AgP comprises a group of severe rapidly progressive forms of periodontitis. It used to be called early-onset periodontitis (EOP), and can be divided into a localised form (previously localised juvenile periodontitis) and a generalised form (previously generalised juvenile periodontitis or generalised EOP). It is characterised by rapid attachment loss and bone destruction. There is no underlying medical condition and usually there is a familial tendency. It often affects young patients, but can occur at older ages as well, hence a cut off age of 35 years is not relevant.

10.28 **Which of the following functions of the predominant inflammatory/immune cells in gingivitis are correct?**

A Plasma cells produce cytokines

B Macrophages produce antibodies

C Macrophages present antigen to lymphocytes

D Macrophages remove damaged tissue

E Polymorphonuclear cells (PMNs) secrete cytokines

10.29 **Which of the following clinical conditions predispose patients with impaired/defective neutrophil function to severe periodontitis?**

A Diabetes mellitus

B Papillon–Lefèvre syndrome

C Ehlers Danlos syndrome

D Chédiak–Higashi syndrome

E Hypophosphatasia

10.30 **Which of the following are appropriate scores and treatment according to the Basic Periodontal Examination (BPE)? The worst results per sextant are included as given below:**

A The coloured band on the probe is completely visible but there is bleeding on probing on a lower right first permanent molar – this would give a score of 3

B The coloured area totally disappears on probing on an upper left second permanent molar – this would give a score of 4

C An overhang on the margin of a restoration on a lower left first permanent molar would give a score of 2

D On probing an upper right central incisor the pocket the coloured area on the probe partially disappears – this would give a score of 3

E The appropriate treatment for BPE score of 3 is oral hygiene instruction (OHI), scaling and root planing

10.28 CDE

Plasma cells produce antibodies and macrophages produce cytokines. PMNs secrete cytokines and inflammatory mediators. They also kill bacteria by intra-cellular and extra-cellular methods.

10.29 ABD

Ehlers Danlos syndrome and hypophosphatasia are associated with abnormal collagen formation, which then leads to periodontal destruction.

10.30 BCDE

The probe used is a World Health Organization (WHO) periodontal probe with a ball end with a diameter of 0.5 mm and a coloured band 3.5–5.5 mm from the tip. The scoring system is shown in the table.

Score	Disease	Treatment
0	No disease	
1	Gingival bleeding, no overhangs or calculus, pockets < 3.5 mm	OHI
2	No pockets > 3.5 mm, subgingival calculus present or subgingival overhangs	OHI, scaling and correction of any iatrogenic factors
3	Pockets within colour-coded area, ie > 3.5 – < 5.5 mm	OHI, scaling and root planning
4	Colour-coded area disappears, pockets > 5.5 mm	OHI, scaling, root planning with or without surgery

10.31 Necrotising gingivitis (necrotising ulcerative gingivitis or NUG):

A   Most commonly affects the first molars

B   Is characterised by interproximal necrosis (tips of papillae)

C   Is commoner in males

D   Is a Gram-positive anaerobic infection

E   Usually produces a characteristic odour

10.32 Management of a patient with NUG may include:

A   20% chlorhexidine mouthwashes twice daily

B   Hydrogen peroxide mouthwash

C   Vigorous toothbrushing

D   Metronidazole 200–400 mg three times daily for 5 days

E   Triamcinolone acetonide (Adcortyl) in Orabase gel applied topically to the lesions

10.33 Which of the following features would suggest that an abscess on a single-rooted tooth was periodontal rather than pulpal in origin?

A   The tooth in question is non-vital

B   The tooth in question is vital

C   There is pain on lateral movement of the tooth

D   There is pain on vertical movement of the tooth

E   There is loss of the alveolar crest height on the radiograph

10.31 BE

Necrotising ulcerative gingivitis most commonly affects the mandibular incisor region and unerupted third molars. There is no predilection for either sex. NUG is a Gram-negative anaerobic infection, and there is usually a foetor-ex-ore, although this is not pathognomic of NUG as it can occur in other pathological conditions of the oral cavity.

10.32 BD

Management of NUG includes removing soft and mineralised deposits in the mouth and improving oral hygiene. However, the lesions are often very painful so patients are not able to use a toothbrush in the initial period. Thus chemical debridement is often used. Mouthwashes such as 0.2% chlorhexidine or hydrogen peroxide are used, as is metronidazole systemically. Triamcinolone acetonide (Adcortyl) in Orobase is a steroid-based preparation that is not indicated for NUG lesions.

10.33 BCE

An abscess originating from the pulp is usually associated with a non-vital tooth, and the tooth is painful on vertical movements. With periodontal abscesses the tooth may be vital and the tooth is painful on lateral movements, and there is often loss of alveolar bone height on radiographs.

10.34 When assessing tooth mobility:

A   Movement of a crown of a tooth in the horizontal plane of less than 0.2 mm is considered normal

B   Grade 1 means movement of the crown of a tooth in the horizontal plane is 0.2–1 mm

C   Grade 2 means movement of the crown of a tooth in the horizontal plane is greater than 1 mm

D   Grade 3 means movement of the crown of a tooth in the horizontal plane is greater than 3 mm

E   Grade 3 means movement of the crown of a tooth in the vertical plane

10.35 Which of the following factors may have a bearing on the measurements recorded on probing pocket depths?

A   The degree of force applied to the probe

B   The thickness of the probe

C   The degree of inflammatory exudate in the gingival soft tissues

D   The bacterial flora in the pocket

E   The amount of gingival crevicular fluid produced

10.36 Regarding dental calculus:

A   It is mineralised dental plaque

B   It is a primary cause of periodontitis

C   The outer surface remains covered by a layer of plaque

D   It is composed of hydroxyapatite

E   It forms when plaque is mineralized from calcium and carbonate ions in the saliva

10.34 ABCE

Tooth mobility is often classified in the following manner:

- Grade 1 – movement of the crown of a tooth in the horizontal plane 0.2–1 mm
- Grade 2 – movement of the crown of a tooth in the horizontal plane greater than 1 mm
- Grade 3 – movement of the crown of a tooth in the vertical plane

10.35 ABC

Periodontal pocket depth probing can be inconsistent due to a number of reasons including: the thickness of the probe; the amount of pressure applied; the angulation of the probe in the pocket; the (mal)position of the probe; and the amount of inflammatory exudate in the soft tissues. The amount of crevicular fluid and the bacterial flora in the pocket do not influence measurement of pocket depths.

10.36 ACD

The primary cause of periodontitis is plaque not calculus. It forms when plaque is mineralised by calcium and phosphate ions in the saliva.

10.37 **A patient attends your practice wearing dentures with a reduced vertical dimension. What complaints may they have due to the reduced vertical dimension?**

A   Difficulty with 'S' sounds

B   Poor appearance showing too little teeth

C   Clicking of teeth when talking

D   Sunken lower face, elderly looking appearance

E   Ill defined pain on the lower denture bearing area that settles when the dentures are removed

10.38 **Which of the following are important to assess before planning treatment that involves an implant-retained lower denture?**

A   History of alcohol intake

B   Oral hygiene

C   Quality of bone

D   Position of maxillary sinus

E   Past history of mouth cancer

10.39 **Which of the following are indications for copy dentures?**

A   To make a spare set of dentures

B   There is a loss of retention, but the rest of the features of the dentures are acceptable

C   Excessive wear of the occlusal surfaces

D   Where the patient lisps

E   Inadequate lip support

10.37   BD

Patients with reduced freeway space often complain of an aged appearance and not showing enough teeth. They may get tired with chewing due to increased masticatory effort being needed. S sounds are not affected by the change in vertical dimension. People wearing dentures with increased vertical dimension often complain of points A, C and E. They may also say that they are 'Showing too much teeth' or their 'Mouth is full of teeth'.

10.38   BCE

A moderate intake of alcohol is not a contraindication for implants but a history of smoking is – as it affects the rate of success of implants. The oral hygiene status and the quality of bone should both be assessed prior to treatment planning. A previous history of mouth cancer is important, in particular, if the patient has received radiotherapy with the risk of osteoradionecrosis. The position of the maxillary sinus is irrelevant.

10.39   ABC

Copy dentures are used to reproduce the favourable aspects of a set of dentures while improving certain features such as occlusion. They are used when patients have had good denture wearing experience with that particular denture. Hence if a patient lisps or there is inadequate lip support some alteration of the polished surfaces of the new dentures would be required.

10.40 Over-dentures:

A   Are contra-indicated in patients with cleft palates

B   Are contra-indicated in patients with inadequate inter-arch space

C   May be indicated when converting a partially dentate patient to a complete denture wearer

D   Are indicated in patients with uncontrolled periodontal disease

E   May be indicated in patients with attrition

10.41 Regarding Kennedy classification for partially edentulous arches:

A   A patient with upper right 8765 and upper left 34567 would be a described as Kennedy Class 4

B   A patient with lower right 54321 and lower left 1234 would be described as Kennedy Class 4

C   A patient with a lower right 76 321 and lower left 123 567 would be described as Kennedy Class 2

D   A patient with a lower right 76 321 and lower left 123 567 would be described as Kennedy Class 3 modification 1

E   A patient with a lower right 87654321 and lower left 123 would be described as a Kennedy Class 3

10.42 Supposed advantages of over-dentures over complete dentures include:

A   Better aesthetics

B   Preservation of alveolar bone

C   The patient will have greater sensory feedback

D   Increased biting forces

E   More reproducible retruded jaw relations

10.40   BCE

Over-dentures are contra-indicated in patients with poor oral hygiene, uncontrolled caries or periodontal disease. There is no reason why a patient with a cleft palate should not have an over-denture and they may be a useful treatment option.

10.41   AD

The Kennedy classification is used to describe partially dentate arches:

- Class 1 – bilateral free end saddles
- Class 2 – one free end saddle
- Class 3 – a unilateral bounded saddle
- Class 4 – a single bounded saddle anterior to the abutment teeth

The classification is based on the most posterior edentulous area, but third molars are not included. A modification, (additional edentulous area), can be added to classes 1–3 when there are other missing teeth. Hence a patient with lower right 54321 and lower left 1234 would be described as Kennedy class 1, a patient with a lower right 87654321 and lower left 123 would be described as a Kennedy class 2.

10.42   BCDE

The aesthetics of complete dentures and over-dentures are comparable. As teeth are retained the patient has greater sensory feedback than when wearing complete dentures. Proprioception is believed to be enhanced and hence there is improved ability to reproduce retruded jaw relations with probable increased chewing thresholds.

10.43 The advantages of immediate dentures are:

A   The existing occlusion can be used for jaw registration purposes

B   The person does not have to be seen without teeth

C   They may act as a haemostatic aid following extractions

D   They usually work out cheaper for the patient

E   They slow down alveolar bone resorption

10.44 Which of the following are potential problems in patients with edentulous maxillae and only lower anterior teeth?

A   Flabby or fibrous upper ridge

B   Anterior seal of upper denture

C   Differential support and retention required in upper denture

D   Lower anterior teeth often worn down because of inadequate vertical height

E   Stability of upper denture

10.45 Surveying of casts for denture design:

A   Is carried out for complete and partial dentures

B   Is only carried out for cobalt-chrome dentures

C   Is used to determine the occlusal vertical dimension

D   Is used to determine undercuts with respect to the path of insertion of a denture

E   Is carried out with the model at right angles to the analyser rod

10.43 ABC

Immediate dentures do have the big psychological advantage that the person does not have to go around without teeth. However, because changes occur in the hard and soft tissues following extraction of teeth the dentures will need adjustment to retain their comfort and fit. This often ends up being more costly as relines need to be carried out or new dentures made. Placing dentures over the alveolar ridges does not reduce bone resorption.

10.44 ACE

Posterior seal of the upper denture is often a problem, as the lower anterior teeth cause the upper denture to tip. There is often over-eruption of the lower anterior teeth causing problems with occlusal plane. The greater force exerted by the natural teeth may lead to flabby ridge formation.

10.45 D

Surveying is carried out to determine undercuts and guide planes and find a path of insertion for a partial denture. It is not used for complete dentures but is carried out for all partial dentures irrespective of construction material.

10.46 Regarding the occlusion of complete dentures:

A   It is desirable to create dentures with canine guidance

B   It is desirable to create dentures with group function

C   It is desirable to create dentures with balanced articulation

D   It is desirable to create dentures with balanced occlusion

E   The occlusion should try to re-create what the patient had naturally

10.47 Regarding partial denture clasps:

A   In order to be functional they must be resisted by a non-retentive clasp arm/component

B   Cast cobalt-chrome clasps need to engage undercuts of greater than 0.25 mm

C   Wrought gold clasps are less flexible than stainless steel clasps

D   The shorter the clasp the more flexible it will be

E   Gingivally approaching clasps are less conspicuous than occlusally approaching clasps

10.48 Regarding connectors in partial dentures:

A   They hold the various parts of the denture together

B   They do not contribute to retention or support of the denture

C   Lingual bars are only used when there is less than 7 mm of space between the floor of the mouth and the gingival margin

D   A sublingual bar is more rigid than a lingual bar

E   Lingual bars are contra-indicated if the lower incisors are proclined

10.46 CD

When constructing complete dentures it is desirable to create both balanced occlusion and balanced articulation. Balanced occlusion means bilateral even contact between the upper and lower dentures in the intercuspal position and balanced articulation means bilateral even contact between the upper and lower dentures in lateral and protrusive movements. This helps maintain the stability of the dentures.

Canine guidance and group function describe the posterior occlusion of the working side teeth during lateral excursions in dentate people. Canine guidance will cause a denture to tip and is not desirable, group function is slightly better, but the ideal is balanced articulation. The patient's natural occlusion is not reproduced in dentures.

10.47 AE

Cast cobalt-chrome clasps need to engage undercuts of less than 0.25 mm as they are stiff and liable to fracture. Wrought gold clasps are more flexible than stainless steel and cast cobalt-chrome clasps, and the longer a clasp is the more flexible it will be.

10.48 AD

Connectors can contribute to support and retention. Lingual bars are only used when there is more than 7 mm of space between the floor of the mouth and the gingival margin, as they need 3 mm clearance from the gingival margin. Lingual bars are contra-indicated if the lower incisors are retroclined.

Index